Bodily Arts

Bodily Arts

RHETORIC AND

ATHLETICS IN

ANCIENT GREECE

❊ ❊ ❊

Debra Hawhee

University of Texas Press, Austin

Requests for permission to reproduce material from this work should be sent to
Permissions, University of Texas Press, P.O. Box 7819, Austin, TX 78713-7819.

⊗ The paper used in this book meets the minimum requirements of
ANSI/NISO Z39.48-1992 (R1997) (Permanence of Paper).

Library of Congress Cataloging-in-Publication Data

Hawhee, Debra.
    Bodily arts : rhetoric and athletics in ancient Greece / by Debra Hawhee.
        p.   cm.
    Includes bibliographical references and index.
        ISBN: 0292721404
    1. Physical education and training—Greece—History—To 1500. 2. Rhetoric,
Ancient. I. Title.
    GV213.H38 2005
    613.7'09495—dc22

                                                                2004005736

This book has been supported by an endowment dedicated to classics and the ancient
world and funded by the Areté Foundation; the Gladys Krieble Delmas Foundation; the
Dougherty Foundation; the James R. Dougherty, Jr. Foundation; the Rachael and Ben
Vaughan Foundation; and the National Endowment for the Humanities. The endowment has also benefited from gifts by Mark and Jo Ann Finley, Lucy Shoe Meritt, the
late Anne Byrd Nalle, and other individual donors.

For J.E.M.

Contents

List of Illustrations

A Note on Texts and Translations

While this book engages classical materials and therefore may be of interest to classicists, I have written it for a broader audience, primarily scholars and students who are interested in the history of rhetoric, rhetorical pedagogy, and studies of the body, and I have therefore tried to make the book accessible to those who do not read classical Greek.

To this end, my quotations of primary ancient materials, unless otherwise noted, follow the latest (widely available and readable) Loeb Classical editions, although I have, for the most part, translated them myself, giving priority to literalness and readability over elegance. At times, however, I have chosen to use others' well-established translations, such as George Kennedy's version of Aristotle's *Rhetoric,* because of its attention to the fine points of rhetoric; and for their energy and beauty, I quote Robert Fagles' editions of the *Odyssey* and the *Iliad,* but with an eye to the Greek and with my own modifications noted.

My transliterations may seem inconsistent, but there is a kind of method to them: for the more widely known proper names, I have used the latinized spelling with which readers will be most familiar. For less familiar names and terms, I use a transliteration of the Greek. I have left some Greek terms (e.g., *agōn, aretē, mētis, kairos*) untranslated, but only after discussing them at some length.

Acknowledgments

One of the points of this book—that knowledge cannot be separated from its conditions of emergence—can be made first, and most explicitly, here in the acknowledgments. Four people in particular served for me as models of learning and figures of discipline and therefore inspire this study most forcefully. They are my *didaskaloi,* Jeffrey Walker and Janet Atwill, and my basketball coaches, Pat Summitt and Larry Ricker. The section on pain's role in bodily learning is lovingly dedicated to Ricker and Summitt, who taught me early on about the diligence involved in learning any kind of art. It was, after all, my not-so-other life as an athlete that put me on this path, and it was Atwill and Walker who kept me there. Their imprints are everywhere, *hapantē.*

My other teachers, too, supported the project from its inception. Sharon Crowley, Richard Doyle, and Cheryl Glenn all differently embody the connection between *philia* and *sophia.* Jeffrey T. Nealon, Evan Watkins, John Muckelbauer, Susan Searls, Dan Smith, Jeremiah Dyehouse, Brad Vivian, and the rhetoricians from the House of Corax, Kakie Urch and J. Blake Scott, all embraced the study enthusiastically and influentially in its early phases.

I am especially grateful for the continuing education I have enjoyed at the University of Illinois. Thanks must go to my Writing Studies colleagues Peter Mortensen, Paul Prior, Cathy Prendergast, and Gail Hawisher. Other colleagues in English and on campus have responded to, talked through, or otherwise inspired parts of the project: Trish Loughran, Julia Walker, and Joe Valente offered intelligent and insightful readings of chapter 7. Julia Saville, Kathie Gossett, Gillen Wood, and

Jim Purdy, perhaps without knowing it, helped spark my interest in the visual. Special thanks to my "body studies" colleagues, Paula Treichler, Alice Deck, Leslie Reagan, C. L. Cole, Bill Kelleher, Andy Orta, Melissa Girard, Jenell Johnson, Scott Herring, Dan Tracy, and (again) Julia Walker and Gail Hawisher, the Illinois Program for Research in the Humanities, and our special guests Jennifer Terry and Leslie Heywood for helping to provide a broad interdisciplinary community. And for general professional encouragement and personal support, Leslea Hlusko, Nancy Castro, Siobhan Somerville, Kal Alston, Zack Lesser, Jed Esty, Stephanie Foote, Cris Mayo, Bill Maxwell, Naomi Reed, and Bob Parker deserve special mention. Special thanks to Amy Wan and Nicole Walls for their help with "endgame" issues.

My cheerful and attentive editors, Andrew Berzanskis and Jim Burr, believed in this book and saw it through. Richard Enos and Takis Poulakos generously provided encouraging and incisive readings of the entire manuscript in its almost-final phases. I hope this newer version can do justice to their suggestions.

The Spencer Foundation provided all-important research networks and fellowship money. Special thanks to my fellow Spencer Fellows Jennifer Kuhn Hanks and Patrick McEwan, and to the awe-inspiring Catharine Lacey. For release time that enabled the manuscript's timely completion, I am grateful to the National Endowment for the Humanities.

My family (Ed, Mary, Dawn, Bill), my friends (Tifani, Rob, Amy, and Regina), and the wee ones (Sarah, Seth, Jada, Sofia, Lucas, Evan, Maggie, and Lola) all emphatically remind me that academia, thankfully, isn't all there is.

And for the innumerable ways they connect to this project and enliven me, I thank, above all, Elizabeth Mazzolini and John Marsh, without whom I would not know the poetics of friendship and love.

D.H.

Champaign, Illinois

31 May, 2003

Bodily Arts

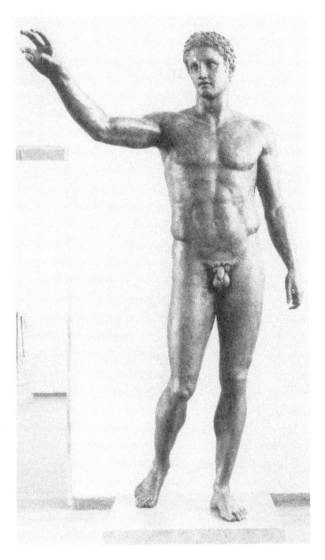

FIGURE I.1
Antikythera Youth, bronze: Athens NM 13396.
© National Archaeological Museum, Athens.

⌗ ⌗ ⌗

Introduction
Shipwreck

Sometime in the first century BCE, a ship destined for Rome, carrying a cargo of Greek sculptures by various artists of the Classical period, went down off the island of Antikythera. For millennia, the shipwreck and its contents remained submerged in the waters of the Ionian Sea, until accidentally discovered by sponge divers in 1901. Found in the cargo was a well-preserved bronze statue of a nude youth (Figure 1), standing 6 feet 4 inches and sporting a broad muscular frame. The statue exhibits a relaxed grace, with the weight resting on the left leg, right arm extending outward, hand holding some sort of round object (now lost).

Aside from speculations about the date and creator of the figure—ranging from the fifth century BCE until Hellenistic times and attributed to various teachers and schools (Hyde 1921: 83)—the major question confounding archaeologists and scholars of ancient sculpture has to do with its identity: what kind of body is this? how might it be classified? is the statue a rendering of god or of mortal? Some believe the statue depicts Perseus holding Medusa's head in his hand, Paris displaying the iconic apple, or Hermes in his role as guardian of the gymnasium.[1] Others read it as an athlete of some sort, perhaps a pentathlete, holding a ball or even a crown or some other prize of victory (Gardner 1903: 152). Still others associate the statue with rhetorical performance, reading the arm as the sweeping, emphatic gesture of an orator (Hyde 1921: 83). Perhaps, such scholars speculate, the statue is Hermes Logios, the god of words, or a mortal rhetor standing on a bema speaking to an assembly.[2]

I begin with this shipwrecked statue not to try to solve the problem of its identity, but rather to introduce a consideration of ancient bodies and bodily arts that would examine the way identity and value circulate through particular bodies as they practice and perform various arts. Such circulation operates, as this book's last chapter suggests, on partner registers of visibility and intelligibility—seeing and recognizing. These registers are most evident in observations like that made by the orator Aeschines, who pointed out that anyone "can recognize an athlete by his bodily vigor (*euexia*) without visiting the gymnasium" (*Against Timarchus* 189). *Euexia,* literally "good bodily disposition," may be located in muscles and sinews as well as in the overall manner of walking, speaking, and carrying oneself, is bound up with the more abstract ancient notion of *aretē,* or virtuosity, to the extent that for the Greeks, such virtuosity inhered in corporeality, inseparable from bodily actions.[3] As Aeschines suggests, then, *euexia* can be recognized— even out of context—if one knows what qualities to look for.

Like Aeschines' wandering athlete, the shipwrecked statue exhibits a readable disposition and manner, a bodily comportment—what the ancients called *hexis.* Yet while the *hexis*-in-action of Aeschines' athlete can be successfully "read" in an associative manner, even outside its expected location (the gymnasium), the dislocation of a shipwreck for a bronzed body is enough to confound modern archaeologists and classical historians. The only certainty is that the statue exhibits a *hexis* that exudes carefully cultivated *aretē* and its associated confident manner. What's more, the shipwrecked statue and the axes of the debates about it—god or mortal? athlete or orator?—suggest a convergence of athletics and rhetoric as arts of *hexis,* in other words, as bodily arts.

The cultural, conceptual, and corporeal connections between the arts of rhetoric and athletics, not unlike the shipwrecked statue, have been more or less submerged since ancient times. To account for this submersion, though, would require a long meditation on disciplinary division, overspecialization, and mind-body separation, all of which this book labors, for the most part, to forget. Such an omission is made possible by the example of the ancient Athenians, to whom strict disciplinary division would have made little sense. In Greece, the Archaic and Classical periods instead marked a time when training was broad, when arts were intricately interwoven, and when mind and body moved and thought together. As such, this book rests on a set of syncretic premises that draw together body and mind; learning and performing; classical studies and rhetorical studies.

Body-Mind

The most explicit link between rhetoric and athletics as arts was made by Isocrates in the mid-fourth century BCE in his treatise *Antidosis*. After claiming that he wants to "begin at the beginning" to describe the emergence of the art of discourse (what he terms philosophy),[4] Isocrates first makes the assertion that humans are naturally made of two parts, body and mind, compounded together, *sugkeisthai* (180). He then goes on to describe how, generations before, certain people,

> seeing many arts (*technas*) established for other things, while none had been arranged for the body and for the mind, invented and left for us double disciplines (*dittas epimeleias*), physical training for the body, of which gymnastics is a part, and, for the mind, philosophy, which I intend to argue are corresponding and united (*antistrophous kai suzugas*) and which, coordinated together (*homologoumenas*), put forward a more intelligent mind and prepare the body to become more useful, not separating by much the two kinds of education, but using similar methods of instruction, exercises, and other forms of discipline. (*Antidosis* 180–83)

In this passage, Isocrates describes a program for shaping a compounded self—body and mind—with training in gymnastics and discourse. Such a program tacitly invokes Plato's program recommending training that balances the body and mind,[5] but Isocrates' program goes further: while Plato calls for a combination of activities that develop the body and that develop the mind, Isocrates notes from the outset a distinctive convergence between these arts.

It is crucial to bear in mind, however, that Isocrates' compounded version of mind-body did not draw together two parts previously separated—Isocrates did not, that is, "blur" the distinction between mind and body or see them as somehow newly interwoven. Such a firm distinction between body and mind is a later development, and we would be remiss to project this perception backward. Ruth Padel frames the problem concisely when she argues that "these critical metaphors of blur and overlap would imply that the Greeks perceived two different things to blur, two meanings to slip between. If the distinctions and meanings are ours, not theirs, then there were no two things for them to blur or be ambiguous about" (1992: 39). At heart, Padel's point is a commentary on method. When thinking syncretically, it is critical to note the places where the arts under consideration are fused together. Whereas these days athletics might function as a metaphor for politics, education, or, in the most clichéd way, for life, I am suggesting that for the ancients, athletics were, at times, all these things together.

Athletics and rhetoric were thus bound together, as Isocrates points out, in at least two ways: 1) unified training in athletics and oratory provides a program for shaping an entire self, and 2) the two arts draw from similar pedagogical strategies wherein the respective instructors impart bodily and discursive forms of expression. Isocrates even joins the arts grammatically in his discussion of pedagogy: "When [the instructors] have made [the students] experienced with these, and they have discussed them with precision, they again exercise the students and habituate them to hard work, and then compel them to combine (*suneirein*) everything they have learned" (*Antidosis* 183–85). Isocrates' model of rhetorical pedagogy therefore works symbiotically with bodily training practices. Not only do the two arts work together to fashion a body-mind complex, they work in a similar way—with parallel rhythms, attention to detail, and broad application.

As this study will demonstrate, then, the linkage in Isocrates' treatise is more than just a clever comparison, and suggests deep relations between rhetoric and athletics, relations that are traceable to Isocrates' forebears, and that were then cultivated and perpetuated by the early sophists and orators in the fifth and fourth centuries BCE. In ancient Athens, athletic and rhetorical practices overlapped and nurtured each other in many ways: culturally, they were founded upon joint values of agonism and *aretē*, and they came together in the ancient festival to combine the visible with the articulable. Pedagogically, they shared modes of knowledge production, an attention to timing, and an emphasis on habituation, imitation, and response. This study will therefore work at the interstices between athletics and rhetoric in order to help elaborate rhetoric's emergence in a network of educational and cultural practices articulated through and by the body.

Learning-Performing

Further inquiry into Isocrates' own syncretism shows that the connections between rhetoric and athletics neither began nor ended with training, but rather emerged from long-time cultural association through agonistic performances in festival and funerary celebrations, associations that carried forward into training practices as rhetoric developed as an art, a *technē*. At the heart of the connection between athletics and rhetoric, then, is an appreciation for the immediate relation between training practices and performance. Because of this shared recognition, these joint arts privilege situated learning and cumulative practice in a chiasmatic way that incorporates performance into learning, learning into performance.

In this regard, the book implicitly enters current conversations in the field of rhetoric and composition, where scholars have long sought to connect pedagogy with performance, particularly in the teaching of writing, the institutional site where contemporary higher education best approximates the ancient treatment of rhetoric as a citizen art. Along these lines, Susan Jarratt's *Re-Reading the Sophists* (1991b) offers an indispensable account of the sophists as teachers and models of particular rhetorical styles. Janet Atwill's monumental study (1998) of Aristotle and the liberal arts raises critical historical questions about liberal values, curriculum, and pedagogy. Takis Poulakos (1997) reads Isocrates as a cultural pedagogue, while Kathleen Welch (1999) uses Isocrates to envision a pedagogy for a technologically saturated culture. These books, all important for figuring rhetoric as a citizen art, provide a critical context for an inquiry attentive to pedagogy as it reaches beyond the classroom.

In addition to works that focus on ancient culture, studies in rhetoric and composition have noticed the usefulness of examining the inventional practices of other arts, the pedagogical value of agonism, the situatedness of learning, and the role of rhythm in learning that this study seeks to elaborate. A few noteworthy studies include Geoffrey Sirc's *English Composition as a Happening* (2002), which figures painting as a possible partner art for writing. Julia Cheville's *Minding the Body* (2001), an ethnographic study of the women's basketball team at the University of Iowa, draws important conclusions about the role of pain (36–37), emotion (51–78), and associative practices in learning. Even more recently, Paul Prior and Jody Shipka (2003) have studied literacy practices as embedded, embodied, rhythmic activities; and Christine Casanave's *Writing Games* (2002) examines the value of agonism and play in improvisational learning, a point also explored in an earlier article by Susan Jarratt (1991b). These works serve as early signs that scholars of rhetoric and composition intuit the imbrication of learning and performance, mind and body, and moreover, that they are beginning to acknowledge how this imbrication can be more easily foregrounded by nontraditional approaches to pedagogy and writing.

Classics-Rhetoric

In addition to allowing an intensive focus on pedagogy and training practices, a syncretism of athletics and rhetoric enables a corollary "thinking together" of classical studies and rhetorical studies. To this end, scholars of classical Greek culture such as J. P. Vernant, Yun Lee Too, Leslie Kurke, Simon Goldhill, John J. Winkler, David Halperin, and Eva Stehle inform these pages just as much as scholars who specialize in the history of rhetoric in speech and English departments— scholars like Jarratt, Atwill, Jeffrey Walker, Richard Leo Enos, Edward Schiappa, James Kastely, Takis Poulakos, and John Poulakos.

Combined with my observation of Isocrates' yoking of rhetoric and athletics, John Poulakos' examination of rhetoric's agonism sparked this inquiry. It was Atwill who introduced me to *mētis* and *kairos* and their relation to the art of rhetoric. Jeffrey Walker's *Rhetoric and Poetics in Antiquity* (2000a), with its examination of rhetoric's emergence in relation to poetic practices, models the kind of deep contextual history this study seeks to produce. Even more recently, Scott Consigny's volume (2001) on the sophist Gorgias suggests that the time is right—*ho kairos estin*—to revisit figures so crucial in rhetoric's development with careful attention to their cultural milieu, historical development, and connections to the arts around them.

As indicated above in the discussion of learning and performing, where rhetoric is linked by discipline with composition and writing studies (usually in English departments), historians of rhetoric often hold special regard for pedagogy as a site for scholarly inquiry. In classics, with the possible exception of George Kennedy's formative early histories of rhetoric, ancient pedagogy has largely been the province of Henri Marrou and Werner Jaegar—until recently. Classical scholar Yun Lee Too has done much to complicate the somewhat monolithic histories put forth by Marrou and Jaegar in the mid-twentieth century. Schooled in contemporary social theory and the vast scholarship on critical pedagogy, Too more precisely parses educational practices in relation to ancient subject production, rather than noting the broad sweeping curricular reforms and movements put forth by Marrou and Jaegar.

Too's earlier books, as examples, focus on identity and subjectivity in relation to Isocrates and ancient pedagogical practices, and her introduction to the recently published *Education in Greek and Roman Antiquity* (2001) makes clear that this work is only the beginning of a detailed reconsideration of ancient pedagogy. While Marrou and Jaegar have done important chronicling work, Too's most recent volume, as she puts it, "acknowledges the social and political dimensions of education in antiquity" (2001: 16), and thus brings contemporary concerns with the politics of pedagogy to bear on ancient artifacts and evidence. That is, Too rightly assumes that education is—and therefore was— political and social: her task in studying the ancients is to find out how this was manifested. In this sense, Too's arguments also inform my turn to ancient athletics and athletic training, for nowhere has athletics been more sociopolitical than in ancient Greece. And nowhere, moreover, as my study argues, has athletics been so intertwined with citizen production.

Similarly, the work of classics and theater scholar Mark Griffith buttresses this book's strong sense that ancient rhetoric and athletics were part of a large network of overlapping practices. Griffith, in an article published in Too's edited volume, observes that educational practices during the Archaic era constitute "a profuse, and often confusing, cluster of institutions and procedures that are usually studied under separate rubrics ... but are probably best considered as one complex, interlocking system" (2001: 36). Such a view, historically warranted, better enables the kind of syncretic work the current book attempts to both perform and recapture.

While Too and Griffith provide important enabling background work, one of the offshoots of viewing different educational practices as part of an "interlocking system" involves the way learning happens, particularly the way it happens corporeally. That is, when viewed in terms of education, rhetoric's relation to athletics hinges on a kind of knowledge production that occurs on the level of the body, displacing the mind or consciousness as the primary locus of learning. Athletic training most clearly exemplifies the role of repetition and imitation in habit production, and the way in which the body takes over in agonistic situations. This is not to say that "mind," or thought, is not important, but rather that it is part of a complex—a mind-body complex—that learns and moves in response to a situation rather than through the application of abstract principles.

In this regard, the study is also informed by a field that can be loosely characterized as "body studies," which includes the work of Judith Butler, Brian Massumi, Michel Foucault, Pierre Bourdieu, and Elizabeth Grosz. These thinkers and others write about the body as a site of torture, affective formation, gender formation, and disciplinary production to consider more precisely the ways in which bodies are bound up with power, identity practices, and learning—in short, the ways in which, to borrow a phrase from Butler, bodies *matter* for philosophical, feminist, even historical inquiry.

Of course, scholars in classical studies and rhetorical studies are noticing bodies as well. As James I. Porter argues in his introduction to *Constructions of the Classical Body,* a concern for the body is neither new nor all that surprising: "On the contrary, the current fascination with the body—its formations, its transformations, and its history—is only the most recent phase and direct consequence of a long *cultivation* of the body in the West. A fascination has, in a way, discovered itself" (1999: 1). Part of this book's aim, then, is to trace the Greeks' role in bodily cultivation, particularly as it relates to the circulation of honor in and through sports and oratory.

Almost simultaneously, rhetorical studies, too, has extended this reflexive fascination with the body and folds it back on rhetoric. The premise of *Rhetorical Bodies* (1999), edited by Sharon Crowley and Jack Selzer, is that rhetoric is articulated through and by bodies, and the work compiles several site-based studies about precisely how such articulation happens in cultural contexts. Similarly, Gail Corning and Randi Patterson's "Researching the Body: An Annotated Bibliography for Rhetoric" (1997) makes quite clear that "the body is no longer simply the province of medical or psychological study" (6). While these two compilations focus on the questions "how are bodies rhetorical?" and "what can body studies do for a consideration of rhetoric?," my study grapples with a slightly different version: How has the body historically functioned as a site of rhetorical production, education, and performance? Tentative answers may be found through an examination of ancient training practices, how they developed, what they were modeled on, and how they would become etched into a classical ethos.

Yet to stop at questions of training would be to miss the critical way that rhetoric as an art of performance functioned in relation to ancient bodies. An examination of this topic guides the book's final chapter, which returns to the notion of identity production. Here, athletic performance, most notably within the context of ancient festivals, emerges as an exemplary locus of honor production, with rhetoric as its necessary supplement, providing the means to articulate and, most important, disseminate honor.

In order to follow rhetoric's movement from cultural values to training practices and back again, the book begins and ends with chapters on the cultural roles and places of athletics and rhetoric in ancient culture. The cultural chapters frame a chain of chapters examining in detail the concepts and practices that bind athletics and rhetoric together: styles of intelligence (*mētis*), immanent, embodied time (*kairos*), the production of one's nature (*phusiopoiesis*), and the space of the gymnasium, which enabled the arts' convergence in the first place.

Chapter 1, entitled "Contesting Virtuosity: Agonism and the Production of *Aretē*," begins by examining the broadly interrelated values of the contest (*agōn*) and virtuosity (*aretē*). The *agōn* was for ancient Athenians the mode of virtue-production *par excellence,* as it provided the occasion for display of ability (*dunamis*) and governed the distribution of glory and honor. Nevertheless, the *agōn* was not entirely about victory—obtaining the prize—but rather invoked notions of "gathering" and "questing." These forces of *agōn* suggest that "questing" after victory—the repetitive engagement in agonistic encounters—was itself a major function of contests. *Aretē* was therefore not entirely outcome-driven, but rather emerged in the encounters themselves, in the act of repeating virtuous actions in relation to others. Chapter 1 delineates these conjoined values and, by doing so, lays the groundwork for an examination of ancient training practices—the mechanisms that shaped the capacity for becoming virtuous.

Chapter 2, "Sophistic *Mētis:* An Intelligence of the Body," examines the ancient notion of *mētis*—cunning intelligence—as an important mode of bodily knowledge production in athletic and sophistic rhetorical training practices. The chapter begins by considering the various figural instantiations of *mētis* in ancient culture—namely the goddess Metis, her progeny Athena, the epic hero Odysseus, and the octopus and fox—and moves on to a reading of Plato's *Sophist,* where the qualities of wily cunning become most explicitly articulated in relation to the figure of the sophist.

Chapter 3, "Kairotic Bodies," extends the treatment of wily intelligence begun in chapter 2 by considering its emergence in particular situations—in response to time as right time, opportunity, occasion, what the ancients termed *kairos.* Once again, *kairos* emerges often in Greek literature and philosophy in the context of athletic and rhetorical encounters—in short, *kairos* is the time of the *agōn,* the immediacy that calls for quick, cunning response. Since so much has been written on the concept of *kairos,* this chapter asks what a particularly athletic notion of *kairos* might bring to a consideration of rhetorical *kairos.* Provisional answers lie in concepts of immanence, movement, embodiment, and the binding together of learning and performing. The chapter moves from the concept itself to the athletic body of the god Kairos as sculpted by Lysippos, to the kairotic practice of Gorgias, whose speeches demonstrate how the concept of *kairos* might work in relation to agonism and bodies. Together, chapters 2 and 3 set the stage for the remaining chapters, as these conjoined concepts of intelligence and immanence call for a situational training, where learning and performing come together most explicitly.

Chapter 4, "*Phusiopoiesis:* The Arts of Training," links *mētis* and *kairos* to training practices by examining the way in which youths were "made ready" for transformation. The chapter develops a term, *phusiopoiesis,* gleaned from a Democritean fragment, to indicate the "production of one's nature." Philosophers and practitioners of ancient medicine—most notably Hippocratic authors, the Presocratics, and Aristotle—all thought a good deal about the nature (*phusis*) of the body and the way in which *phusis* can be rendered malleable, made (*poiei*) into something else. The chapter then moves into a delineation of the various dynamics of ancient *phusiopoiesis*—the cultivation of a readiness, friendship, provocation, the matrices of pain and erotics—all of which formed a network of relational, productive practices between student and teacher, or self and other.

This network of productive practices becomes a primary area of inquiry for the next two chapters. Chapter 5, "Gymnasium I: The Space of Training," offers an analysis of the ancient gymnasium with attention to the way spatial distribution facilitated a kind of gathering that made the area ripe for infiltration by sophists and philosophers alike. Pierre

Bourdieu's notion of *habitus,* a system of dispositions that emerge in relation to structures and practices, offers a useful way to conceptualize the interaction between space and habit formation—between the dynamics of *phusiopoiesis* and the traffic between athletic and rhetorical training in the ancient gymnasium, the locus for citizen training.

Chapter 6, "Gymnasium II: The Bodily Rhythms of Habit," extends the spatial analysis into mechanisms of habit formation by discussing sophistic pedagogy in terms of its "3Rs." The "3Rs" of sophistic education were not content-based, as 3Rs are now construed; rather, the main components of sophistic training have to do with a manner, a habituated style of thought and action: rhythm, repetition, and response. The gymnasium had a rhythm all its own, often established by pipe players, who provided musical accompaniment for gymnastic and rhetorical exercises.

Here, music's direct role in shaping one's *ēthos*—character or disposition—becomes critical for a consideration of transformative training practices. Athletic and rhetorical training practices also incorporated repetition to enable rhythmic movements to become ingrained in one's body. From such attentive, repetitive, rhythmic practice, in imitative or agonistic relation to someone or something else, emerges a pedagogy of response, as students develop the capacity to respond to singular situations. Put simply, the best training for the *agōn* is the *agōn,* the repeated production of encounters with others.

Chapter 7, "The Visible Spoken: Rhetoric, Athletics, and the Circulation of Honor," thus returns to the *agōn,* this time to the contest between rhetoric and athletics as arts of existence. The chapter considers the ways in which the orators Isocrates and Demosthenes explicitly struggle with how to use the *aretē*-saturated milieu of athletics to help establish rhetoric's own importance as a worthwhile and honorable art. At issue in this inquiry is the tangled relation between visibility and articulability—between the production of honor at the bodily level, as in the case of athletic victors, and the re-production of that same honor in rhetorical commemorations of the event, tales of the feat, rumors of greatness. The Athenians, honor-loving humans that they were, greatly admired their heroic athletes, but it was rhetoric—discourse about this very honor-love conjunction (*philotimia*)—that enabled and sustained honor's circulation.

This study, by drawing together rhetoric and athletics, thus simultaneously draws together classics and rhetoric; learning and performing;

mind and body. Such a syncretic approach shifts attention away from questions of rhetoric's origin and development to questions of the conditions of rhetoric's emergence, which was bound up in an interactive struggle of sociocultural forces. As such, it allows a perspective on rhetoric as an art that was deeply situated in Greek culture and entangled with other arts of subject production. A focus on rhetoric's connections to athletics enables a view of rhetoric as a bodily art rather than strictly a cerebral endeavor, and traces the way in which rhetoric and athletics mutually shaped and struggled with each other—conceptually, practically, and culturally.

❄ 1 ❄

Contesting Virtuosity

Agonism and the Production of *Aretē*

The role of the *agōn,* the struggle or contest, in early Greek culture cannot be overemphasized: it was the place where wars were won or lost (or, for that matter, happened at all), the reason gods and goddesses came into being, the context for the emergence of philosophy and art, and even, according to Hesiod, the reason crops grew (*Works and Days* 11ff.). In the name and spirit of the *agōn,* bodies not only came together, they *became* bodies, bodies capable of action and (hence) identity formation. This chapter will focus on the notion of agonism as a dynamic through which the ancients repeatedly produced themselves, and which functioned as a point of cultural connection between athletics and rhetoric.

It must be stressed from the outset that the *agōn* is more than the one-on-one sparring that is emphasized in most treatments of the topic. That is, agonism is not merely a synonym for competition, which usually has victory as its goal. For outcome-driven competition, the Greeks used the term *athlios,* from the verb *athleuein,* meaning to contend for a prize. The *agōn,* by contrast, is not necessarily as focused on the outcome as is *athlios,* the more explicit struggle for a prize. Rather, the root meaning of *agōn* is "gathering" or "assembly" (*LSJ*). The Olympic Games, for example, depended on the gathering of athletes, judges, and spectators alike. *Agora,* the marketplace, shares the same derivation and a strikingly similar force of meaning as *agōn,* and, as is commonly known, functioned as the ancient gathering place *par excellence.* Whereas *athlios* emphasizes the prize and hence the victor, *agōn* emphasizes the event of the gathering itself—the contestive encounter rather than strictly the division between opposing sides.

To be sure, however, the "gathering" force of *agōn* to some extent entails—and is enabled by—victory. An aim of this exploration, though, is less to consider agonism's teleological, victory-driven side, and more to foreground the agonistic encounter itself. For rhetoric, this encounter-gathering side of *agōn* constitutes the more pervasive agonal dynamic; it is this dynamic that figures prominently in the shape of rhetoric's agonism, and, by extension, its status as a bodily art.

John Poulakos' important book on the sophists (1995) points out the agonistic connection between rhetoric and athletics (32–39), arguing that the sophists effectively "turned rhetoric into a competitive enterprise" (35) and that athletics provided a "rich vocabulary" for the rhetorical art. Poulakos' account, however, focuses on the *athlios* side of agonism, the "victory at all cost" mentality. Yet the "gathering" force of the *agōn* inheres in rhetoric as well, most obviously in the very structure of rhetorical situations and their dependence on an assembly, but also in the training and production of a rhetorical subject. The realm of training, further, shows most clearly the close relation between *athlios* and *agōn,* as a drive for the prize depends on agonistic logic from the very beginning.

Agōn is also connected with the verb *agein,* which is generally translated "to lead," but in some instances is linked to training and can be translated "to bring up, train, educate" (e.g., Plato, *Laws* 782d). So the word *agōn* can suggest movement through struggle, a productive training practice wherein subject production takes place through the encounter itself. As Nietzsche observes, the Greeks produced themselves through active struggle; their pedagogy depended on agonism (1974b: 58).

Taking seriously rhetoric's emergence in the context of the *agōn* requires a reconfiguration of rhetoric as an agonistic encounter. That is, for the sophists at least, agonism produces rhetoric as a gathering of forces—cultural, bodily, and discursive—thus complicating the easy portrayal of rhetoric as *telos*-driven persuasion (i.e., persuasion with a specific end) or as a means to reach consensus. Further, the emergence of agonistic rhetoric and its relationship to virtuosity was enabled by the agonistic force of athletics. As a result, the sophistic rhetorical exemplar was the athlete in action. Perhaps the stranger in Plato's *Sophist* said it best when he dubbed the typical sophist "an athlete in the contest of words" (*agōnistikēs peri logous ēn tis athlētēs*) (231e). I will argue, then, that it was a peculiarly athletic notion of agonism—one that balances the gathering and combative meanings—that functioned as an important molder of early rhetorical practice and pedagogy.

"A Politics of Reputation"

A treatment of the agonistic link between rhetoric and athletics requires a corollary consideration of *aretē*, a kind of virtuousness that in its own way drove agonistic encounters, as Greeks sought after the esteem of others through competitive engagement and display of their abilities, be they skill at javelin throwing or delivery of an encomium.

Since "*aretē*" is so complex and difficult to render in English, I will often simply render it as *aretē;* my use of the term "virtuosity," however—rather than its typical translation as "virtue"—signals the concept's status as a condition the ancients repeatedly tried to achieve, a condition not unrelated to art and skill. Virtuosity, then, is meant to stand apart from contemporary notions of "virtue" that teeter on the edge of moralizing. *Aretē*, that is, was an ethical concept, and as such was associated with bodily appearance, action, and performance as much as it was conceived of as an abstracted "guide" for such actions.

Thus at the heart of the ancient *agōn* lies the concept of *aretē*, for the struggling contest served as a stage of sorts. Early on *aretē* was associated with the goodness, courage, and prowess of a warrior. One of the best examples of early agonistic manifestations of *aretē* can be found in Homer's Achilles, who is referred to as "strong," "swift," and "godlike" (1.129; 1.140); "the great runner" (1.224); and "the best of the Achaeans" (16.279). Achilles' *aretē* has a double force, for not only is he a brave and brilliant warrior, but from the outset he is destined to die in battle at Troy (1.536) with the utmost glory, a guarantor of *aretē*. Conceptually, *aretē* was tightly bound with *agathos* (goodness), *kleos* (glory), *timē* (honor), and *philotimia* (love of honor).

As David Cohen points out, the norms and practices of Athenian virtuosity "operate within the politics of reputation, whose normative poles are honor and shame" (1991: 183). As such, *aretē* functions as an external phenomenon, depending on forces outside the "self" for its instantiation. *Aretē* thus operated within an economy of actions, wherein certain acts, such as dying in battle or securing a victory at the Olympic Games, were considered *agathos* and hence deserving of honor, and certain acts were not. In other words, one cannot just *be* virtuous, one must become virtuosity itself by performing and hence embodying virtuous actions in public. *Aretē* was a critical function of *agōn:* not a *telos,* but rather a constant call to action that produced particular habits. In short, virtuous movements produced a repeated *style* of living—the economy of *aretē* was a decidedly bodily phenomenon.

For ancient Athenians, identity did not precede actions, and this applied to all aspects of one's life. That is, one could not just "be" manly (*andreios*) and all that entails without displaying "manliness" through manly acts of courage. In the *Iliad,* an epic primarily concerned with human achievement, the outside—the place from which commendations come—can be located with the Olympian gods. In Homeric epic the gods serve as arbiters of glory, or *kleos,* acting not just as approving judges, but as the very enablers of heroic actions.

In this regard, the interventions of Athena are telling. In Book 5 of the *Iliad,* Athena guides the spear of Diomedes into Pandaros' face (290–91) and then into Ares' midsection (856–57), and in Book 23, Athena trips Ajax in a footrace (774–75), thus sealing Achilles' victory. As Seth L. Schein notes, such interventions say less about the agency of the gods versus humans and more about the goodness of the hero receiving assistance from the gods. That is, as Schein puts it, "the presence of the god was the traditional poetic means of calling attention to the greatness of the victor and the victory, and it likewise conferred a special dignity on both victor and victim by showing that the gods themselves were concerned to intervene in their struggle" (1984: 58). So the very notion that a god or goddess would care to intervene suggests that honor is at stake and that, in the context of Homeric epic, the gods function as exterior forces in charge of conferring *kleos.* The resulting actions—the slicing of Pandaros' face and Achilles' winning of the footrace—are deemed indicators of virtuosity by the onlookers in the poem as well as its readers/listeners.

Establishing oneself as a great warrior and dying in battle were of course not the only ways to achieve fame in ancient Greece. As the example of Achilles' footrace suggests, the "politics of reputation" also operated in athletic competitions, sometimes held as part of funerary rituals (as in the *Iliad* and the *Odyssey*) and sometimes as part of celebratory festivals, as is the case with the Isthmian, the Pythian, the Nemean, and the Olympic Games. Much like the warrior Achilles, athletes relied on and responded to "the outside" (opponents, spectators, judges) as witnesses and conferrers of *aretē*. Of course, the *agōn's* emphasis on response in the moment troubles the very notion of an "outside," for the relational quality of struggle makes opponents, spectators, and judges part of a network of agonistic production.

Corporeality, Virtuosity

A common way to memorialize athletes and other famed men was to erect statues in their name. For the victorious athlete, not only did the statue-form function as a mark of *aretē*, but its carefully crafted surface also served to simulate virtuosity, to radiate *aretē* from its rendering of bodily parts (limbs, abdomen, ears, eyes, etc.). In other words, statues, like the victorious athletes they commemorated, invoked, embodied, and hence modeled *aretē* for their beholders.

For ancient Athenians, physical beauty and moral superiority were inextricably tied (Vernant 1989: 28–29). This double force of *aretē* is suggested by the phrase for nobility, *kalos kagathos,* "the beautiful and good." Delineator that he is, Aristotle parses the beautiful, the good, and *arēte* as follows: "now *kalon* describes whatever, through being chosen for itself, is praiseworthy or whatever, through being good [*agathon*], is pleasant because it is good [*agathon*]. If this then, is the *kalon,* then *aretē* is necessarily *kalon;* for it is praiseworthy of being good [*agathon*]" (*Rh.* 1366a; trans. Kennedy). Aristotle's description of these qualities points to their indissoluble connections: *kalos, agathos,* and *arēte* relate recursively, almost tautologically, each standing as evidence for the other.

Furthermore, this passage sketches *kalos kagathos* as an outwardly projected quality, a decidedly corporeal feature: here, "the pleasant" entails that which is enjoyed because it is exhibited by one and experienced by others. Jean-Pierre Vernant, keen on the body's role in exhibiting *kalos kagathos,* writes,

> The Greek body of Antiquity did not appear as a group morphology of fitted organs in the manner of an anatomical drawing, nor in the form of physical particularities proper to each one of us, as in a portrait. Rather, it appears in the manner of a coat of arms and presents through emblematic traits the multiple "values" — concern-

ing his life, beauty and power with which an individual is endowed, values which he bears and which proclaim his *timē*, his dignity and rank. (1989: 28)

Such "emblematic" traits, distinctive markers of *aretē*, often invoke the bodies of the gods, what Vernant designates "divine superbodies," bodies that radiate splendor.[1] Vernant also points out that images of men engaging in athletic activity exhibit "stature, breadth, presence, speed of leg, strength of arm, freshness of complexion, and a relaxation, suppleness and agility of limbs" (28). These qualities, along with their suggestion of a capacity for the *agōn*, for the frenetic battle, "can be read upon [the body] like marks that attest to what a man is and what he is worth" (28). Such marks constituted a corporeal code of *aretē*.

Along these same lines, in the *Rhetoric*, Aristotle designates the following as features of "virtuosity of the body" (*sōmatos aretas*): "health, beauty, strength, physical stature, athletic prowess" (1360b4; trans. Kennedy). Later he elaborates "bodily *aretē* in competition (*agōnistikē de sōmatos aretē*)" as follows:

> a combination of size and strength and swiftness (and swiftness is actually a form of strength); for one who can throw his legs in the right way and move quickly and for a distance is a runner, and one who can squeeze and hold down is a wrestler, and one who can thrust the fist is a boxer, and one who can do both of the latter two has the skills needed for the *pankration*, and one who can do them all [has the skills] for the pentathlon. (1361b14; trans. Kennedy)

Noteworthy in this passage is the way in which bodily features become discrete and recognizable actions or capacities (*dunamenos*). Identities are thus inseparable from potential movements: one who is able to execute a certain type of "hold" is a wrestler, for example. Capacities (*dunameis*) can be suggested by particular bodily features, and this is where *kalos* becomes important. Aristotle observes that for youth, beauty "is a matter of having a body fit for the race course and ordeals of strength, pleasant to look at for sheer delight; thus pentathletes are the most beautiful because they are equipped by nature at one and the same time for brawn and for speed" (1361b11; trans. Kennedy). The "equipment" for strength and speed, probably suggested by an even bodily distribution of moderate musculature, is then linked directly to beauty, which, as Aristotle points out only a few lines later, signals aretē: "*aretē* is necessarily *kalon*."

There is apparently no need for Aristotle to describe the particular ways in which strength and brawn manifest themselves corporeally, for *kalos* invokes an already established ideal. As Vernant puts it, "the category of the body is less a matter of precisely determining its general morphology or the particular form nature gives to one individual or another than it is a matter of situating the body between the opposite poles of luminosity and darkness, beauty and ugliness, value and foulness" (1989: 31–32). Aristotle upheld the body of the athlete as one which most closely approximates *kalos kagathos,* and this identity was secured in the particular capacities marked most notably by bodily configurations or in the stylized movements of the athletic body. Bodily *aretē* thus aligns with corporeal capacity, signs of work and development quite literally built up in the body through training for particular movements.

The body's appearance of work and development then exhibits virtuosity, for in ancient Greece, one *is* what one *does,* a point that James Redfield argues in his exploration of Homeric culture and values. "Homeric man," he argues, exists on an outward plane, constituted only by his surface: "such a man is not an enclosed identity; he is rather a kind of open field of forces . . . there is no clear line for him between *ego* (I) and *alter* (other)" (1994: 21). Though distinctly Homeric according to Redfield, this constitution by the outer or outside still persisted in the fourth century, as evidenced by Aristotle's treatment of the surface-quality of *kalos kagathos* and the correspondence between *aretē* and actions.

The link between action and identity is also emphasized by the Olympian gods, each of whom inhabited a particular domain of identity-producing action. Not surprisingly, then, the gods most connected to athletics sported the most bodily *aretē* and were imitated by the sculptors of athlete statues. Apollo, Hermes, and Heracles all functioned as gods of contests, and their forms were evoked by athletic statues (Hyde 1921: 100–109). Statues were fashioned on a visual logic of such godlike forms, hence the confusion about the identity of the shipwrecked statue with which this study began.

Characteristics of *aretē* thus included glory, honor, courage, and bodily strength and swiftness to succeed in battle. As Joseph M. Bryant points out, mythical and historical warriors served as *paradeigmata,* or exemplars, of outward, bodily excellence (1996: 28). These ideals, of course, were incorporated into educational practices in the form of military and athletic training (see also Marrou 1956: 36–40). The somatic *ethoi* of athlete and warrior were thus tightly bound in Hellenic culture: both exhibited the bodily excellence of strength in their muscled physiques, which were suggestive of the capacity (*dunamis*) for actions exhibiting courage and honor.

If their bodies so unmistakably radiated *aretē,* what, then, distinguished athletes and warriors from gods? The answer, it seems, is the necessity of the *agōn*—the battle or contest—to actualize the capacity for virtuosity and thereby affirm the presence of *aretē:* while divine somatic *aretē* stood as evidence for itself, bodily *aretē* had to be enacted repeatedly in the case of mortal athletes or warriors. For this repetitive enactment, the *agōn* was *aretē*'s stage. As such, the *agōn* was central to the production of *aretē,* or the complex aggregate of bodily and conceptual attributes—honor, glory, excellence—which I will call the "Olympic ethos." Olympic here suggests multiple forces at work in the production of this ethos. First, there is "Olympic" writ large—strong in body and large in *aretē.* Next, Olympic relates to the Olympian gods, who, as evidenced in the *Iliad,* functioned as arbiters of *kleos* as well as exemplars of *aretē* themselves. Finally, Olympic ethos invokes the Olympic Games, the primary and most widely regarded of agonal scenes in Greece, which, of course, were necessarily tied to the gods in name and tribute.

The Olympic ethos became a defining trait of Hellenic culture. As paragons of this culture, heroes, warriors, and athletes did not fade with time. The founding of the Olympic Games in 776 BCE is politically most significant as the first "pan-Hellenic" event and is hence commonly used to mark Greek chronology, as events are noted according to the "Olympiad" in which they occurred. The year 776 is also commonly designated as the beginning of the Archaic period in Greece, the period, as Bryant and Burkert both suggest (Bryant 1996: 80–84; Burkert 1985: 105–7), dominated by "agonal man," producer and bearer of the Olympic ethos delineated above; a similar logic persists as well in the cultural production of Pericles as "the Olympian" (de Romilly 1992: viii; Plutarch, *Lives* 8.2). At the heart of the ancient relationship between *aretē* and agonism is the very logic for linking rhetoric and athletics.

"Questing" for *Aretē:* Pindar's Victory Odes and the *Agōn*

In order to track *aretē* back to the agonal dynamic with which this chapter started, I will delineate the Olympic ethos by pursuing the athletic *agōn* a bit further.

Along with sculpture, poetry served as a means of conferring and reproducing athletes' virtuosity, but poetic depictions of athletes produce *aretē* with a slightly different force than did athlete-statues.[2] While the bronze and marble muscles render *aretē* in terms of bodily capacity, the discursive rendering of athletes in poetry elaborates the quality and magnitude of the Olympic ethos emerging from success in competition.

The Olympic ethos is spotlighted most notably in the odes of Pindar, the fifth-century epinician poet. While sculptures of athletes by their very constitution offer a pedagogy of virtuous corporeal codes, Pindar's *epinikia* (poems commemorating a victory) offer a pedagogy of the movements of virtuosity that occur in the context of agonal festivals. Indeed, for Pindar, virtuosity is nothing but particular styles of movement. As Pindar put it, "far shines that fame of Olympic festivals . . . where competition is held for swiftness of feet and boldly laboring feats of strength" (*Ol.* 1.92–96; trans. Race). What's more, Pindar's second *Olympian Ode* suggests that victory (*nikē*) is not necessarily the sole proof of *aretē,* but rather a symptom of becoming virtuous. He sings, "Winning releases from anxieties one who engages in competition. Truly, wealth embellished with *aretais* provides fit occasion for various achievements by supporting a profound and questing pursuit (*merimnan agroteran*)" (52–55). Here, the word translated as "questing" (*agroteron*) in its nominal form denotes hunter or huntress, the one who is "fond of the chase" (*LSJ*). Victory, in combination with wealth and other virtuous actions, indexes such a questing, as it marks a continual pursuit of virtuosity. What matters for *aretē* then, is not the victory per se but rather the hunt for the victory.

"Questing," for Pindar, necessarily entails certain risks and much work, as he writes in an ode for the winner of the mule race at Olympia in 472/468 BCE: "Achievements without risk win no honor among men or on hollow ships, but many remember if a noble deed is accomplished with toil" (*Ol.* 6.9–12; trans. Race). The emphasis on the quest rather than on the victory itself is consistent throughout Pindar's *epinikia*. Take, for example, his tribute to Hagesidamos, the winner of boys' boxing in 476 BCE, into which Pindar incorporates a general comment on the Olympic Games:

> Time moved forward and declared the plain truth:
> how Heracles divided up the gift of war and offered the choice
>   part,
> and how he established the four years' festival with the first
>   Olympic Games
> and its victories.
> Who then won the new crown
> with hands or feet or chariot,
> after fixing in his thoughts the boast
> of the contest and achieving it in deed? (*Ol.* 10.55–63)

Pindar goes on to list early victors in running, wrestling, and box-ing—that is, those who fixed their thoughts on an achievement and emerged from the contest as victors. But the focus here is the very act of "fixing in his thoughts" (*doxa themenos*). The gerundive *themenos* comes from the multivalent *tithēmi,* which can have the force of placing or de-positing, as well as executing and producing. *Themenos* thus invokes the productive force of "setting one's mind" to something, which is most— if not all—of the game, according to Pindar. At the very least, it is the act of "fixing" one's mind to virtuosity, and the concomitant "questing" that is the most suggestive of agonal glory for Pindar.

In many ways, Pindar's encomiastic art demands a narrative of on-going, repeated production. *Aretē,* that is, cannot be something that one merely happens upon by chance, or it would become difficult to cele-brate as a remarkable achievement. As Hesiod had long before pointed out, there has to be sweat before *aretē* (*Works and Days* 289; Vernant 1983: 252).

In this context, then, *agōnes* provided occasions for showcasing the effects of one's "questing." It is important here once again to distin-guish between the actions during the contests and the prizes won by vic-tors. While the agonistic performance—the actual athletic movements —demonstrated *aretē,* the prizes (*athlioi*) were more closely aligned with *kleos* (glory or fame). This subtle distinction becomes apparent in *Isthmian* 1, where Pindar sings of the athletes Kastor and Iolaos:

> and in athletic games (*aethloisi*) they attempted the most contests
>   (*pleistōn agōnōn*),

and adorned their houses with tripods,
cauldrons, and bowls of gold,
tasting (*geuomenoi*) the crowns of victory.
Their virtue (*areta*) shines (*lampei*) clearly
in the naked footraces and in the hoplite races with clattering
    shields.
Just as in their hands as they fling javelins
and when they hurl the stone discuses. (18–25)

The first part of this passage points to the prizes awarded to victors,
and the verb *geuomenoi*, a middle form of *geuō*, suggests that athletes
"taste" victory and its attendant *kleos*, thus implying that they nourish
their craving for the prize, the end of victory. Importantly, however, it is
during the *agōn* itself, in the bodily movements of the athlete, and not in
the gleaming cauldrons or bowls, that *aretē* becomes conspicuous. The
outward movement or enactment of *aretē* in the hurling of the javelin
stands in distinction to the inward-movement of glory back toward the
athlete at the contest's end. The *agōn* is thus sutured to *aretē* insofar as
athletes are engaged in their quest for virtuosity with an eye to the contests or gatherings where their arduous efforts would be acknowledged
and potentially rewarded.

What's more, the naked footraces and clattering shields suggest that
the economy of *aretē* is decidedly corporeal, material, and active.
Again, in the same way that warriors continually exhibited virtuosity,
athletes competed over and over, suggesting that the "questing," the
training for and performing of excellent actions—not merely the victory—repeatedly produced *aretē*.

Agonism

If questing was foremost in the production of *aretē* and it was the struggle involved in questing that really mattered, it is important to delineate the precise character of that struggle. Indeed, it is the idea of the
struggle or strife that fascinated and drove the ancients, starting at least
in Homeric times. The idea of productive strife as a principle of movement is central, for example, to Hesiod's *Works and Days,* where he delineates two kinds of strife:

There was not only one race of Strife (*eridōn*), but over the earth
there are two. On the one hand, there is that which a man would

praise when he came to apprehend it; but on the other hand there is that which is blameworthy. Their spirit is divided. The one is bound to evil war and battle: it is abominable; no mortal loves it, but by necessity they honor the heavy Strife according to the plans of the gods. The other gloomy Night brought forth first, and so the son of Cronus, who sits above and resides in the ether, placed it in the roots of the earth and made it much better for men. This kind of strife rouses a man to work even if he is shiftless. For, if a person without work in hand sees another, a wealthy man who hurries to plow and plant and put his house in good order, then that neighbor envies his neighbor who hurries after riches. This is the good Strife for mortals: potter is angry with potter and carpenter with carpenter; beggar envies beggar, and singer, singer. (Hesiod, *Works and Days* 11–26)

Hesiod's concern is primarily with the effects of the two kinds of strife. While one kind of strife can be destructive insofar as it manifests itself in war resulting in death (among other things), the other kind of strife can be productive, placing people in relation to land, to plants, to each other, and producing struggles on many levels. In the context of *Works and Days,* "good strife" rouses (*egeirei*) men and makes them hurry (*speudei*), thus making them more efficient land workers. The Greek word used for strife here is a derivation of *eris,* generally translated as strife, quarrel, contention, or discord; *eris* later became closely allied in meaning with *agōn,* a contest (*LSJ*), and with our "eristics," disputation.

While overshadowed in contemporary uses of the term by the destructive, "takeover," teleological force (as in CBS Sports' "'agony' of defeat"), the productive quality of agonism delineated by Hesiod nevertheless still inheres in contemporary pharmacological research, where agonism is a key concept in drug-cell relations. This relatively recent instantiation of the word is instructive, for its contemporary meanings actually help illustrate more precisely what I take to be Hesiod's distinctions. In pharmacodynamic language, the term "agonism" designates the bonding of a drug chemical with what is termed a receptor, a special area on the outer surface of the cell membrane. The agonistic bonding then triggers a change in cellular activity. In other words, agonism denotes an encounter, the production of a response, and a subsequent change in both substances.

By contrast, a drug that produces the opposite effect—i.e., blocking a receptor or inhibiting response—is termed an antagonist (Graham 1979: 15–16). The notion of antagonism is crucial for understanding the forces of agonism. Whereas antagonism blocks a response, agonism, by definition, demands one. The *agōn* is thus constituted by a modality of response, the production of some kind of movement, be it a speeding up or slowing down, of cell activity—in pharmacological terms—or of discursive or bodily activity, in other terms. Because it depends upon molecular affinity (Kenakin 1993) for response production, agonism can be delineated as a response-producing encounter.

Contemporary pharmacological terminology thus preserves the distinction between antagonism and agonism evident in Hesiod's delineation of destructive and productive strife. On one hand, antagonism (or destructive strife) is characterized by stoppage of movement or death, as in war. Agonism, on the other hand, produces envy and speed in movement. As Vernant contends, Hesiod's passage valorizes "a life of mixtures" (1983: 20). This agonistic movement, or "life of mixtures," described in *Works and Days* invokes notions of excellence that are prominent in the Homeric poems, where the *agōn* offers an occasion for the demonstration and hence production of virtuosity.

Rhetoric, the Sophists, and *Logōn Agōnes*

If the athletic *agōn* most vividly displays bodily *aretē,* then the rhetorical *agōn* may draw on this same mode of display by invoking the similarities between the two venues. In fact, rhetoric and athletics often shared the same venue, festivals: the sophist Gorgias was, according to Philostratus, "conspicuous (*emprepōn*) also at the festivals of the Greeks" (DK 82 A1). Philostratus mentions the Pythian festival, and Pausanias points out that Gorgias "was famous for the speeches he gave at the Olympic Games" (DK 82 A7). Gorgias is also said to have spoken at Olympic festivals robed in purple (Aelian, *Misc. History* 12.32; DK 82 A9). Executing the logic of dazzling display, his robe and eloquence created an equivalence between his art and that of the famed Olympic wrestlers, prompting Diodorus Siculus to observe centuries later that Gorgias was "in the power of speech by far the most eminent of the men of his time" (DK 82 A4). A poetic precursor of the cultural joining of Gorgias with athletes may be found in Pindar's *Olympian* 1, where the athlete/leader (Hieron) stands together with the poet (Pindar) on the "summit" of achievement (lines 111–15).[3]

The questing aspect of agonism (and its connection to *aretē*) carried over into other modes of training and performance, as the *agōn* and its attendant Olympic ethos permeated the realms of drama, poetry, and music. It is therefore not surprising that sophistic discursive practices and ideas about an orator's virtuosity emerged within the agonal scene as well, and that a questing component was similarly inserted into rhetorical pedagogy. According to Diogenes Laertius, Protagoras was among the first to join competition and rhetoric, for he was responsible for the inception of competitive debates—*logōn agōnes* (80 A1 52).

Moreover, the sophists, particularly Protagoras, held wide repute for their controversial claim of teaching *aretē* to young men. Plato, for example, depicts Protagoras making the following assertion in the dialogue bearing his name: "I have shown you by both myth and argument (*logon eirēka*) that *aretē* is teachable (*hōs didakton aretē*)" (328c).[4] Not unlike Pindar, for the sophists, questing after *aretē* and the related repetitions of virtuous actions were what constituted and/or produced virtuosity.

In the same dialogue, the young Hippocrates expresses an interest in entering into regular conversations, *sunousia,* with Protagoras.[5] The character Protagoras describes his educational philosophy to Hippocrates as follows: "Young man, you will gain this by joining my conversations, that on the day when you join them you will go home a better man, and on the day after it will be the same; every day you will constantly improve more and more" (318a–b). It is thus through the repeated act of attempting to perform *aretē* via regular encounters with Protagoras, day after day—as in Pindar's questing—that one achieves virtuosity.

That the sophists incorporated agonism into their art is one of the few extant certainties about this group of thinkers and teachers. Indeed, Timon called the old sophist "Protagoras[,] who mixes in (*epimeiktos*), master of wrangling (*erizemenai eu eidōs*)" (DK 80 A1 52). The word *epimeiktos* suggests one who resides in combination with others and comes from the verb *epimeignumi,* which has various aspects, including "to add by mixing," "to mingle with others," and "to have intercourse." All these dimensions of *epimeiktos* suggest that Protagoras' teachings fostered a mode of relation and response, thus tapping into the "gathering," response-provoking force of the *agōn* discussed above.

Protagoras' *logōn agōnes* emerged from the idea of the contest, most accessible in the form of combat sports like wrestling, boxing, and the pankration, a more violent combination of wrestling and boxing. And the effects of a sophistic *agōn* were apparently much like those of an athletic contest, as Socrates narrates one such encounter with Protagoras: "His speech really produced noise and approval from many of the listeners; and at first I felt as though I had been struck by a skillful boxer, and was quite blind and dizzy with the effect of his words and their shouts of approval" (*Protagoras* 339e). It is worth noting, too, that in this particular instance, Socrates and Protagoras wrangle to an inconclusive draw and part respectfully.

The agonistic impulse was also alive in Gorgias' bold challenge to the audience to "name a subject" on which he would discourse. The sophist Hippias made a similar promise to "speak on whatever subject anyone may choose from those I have prepared for a display, and to answer whatever question anyone may wish to ask," but Hippias added an extra hint of self-assurance: "For never, since I began to compete (*agōnizesthai*) at Olympia, have I met anyone superior to myself in anything" (DK 86 A8).[6]

Here, Hippias refers to competitions in oratory, held as part of Olympic festivals, in which he and Gorgias were reputed to have taken part.[7] Although Protagoras was known as the father of these debates, Gorgias too was remembered in connection with the *agōn*, as evidenced in this epigram inscribed on a statue base at Olympia dating back to the beginning of the fourth century:

No one of mortals before discovered a finer art
Than Gorgias to train (*askēsai*) the soul for contests of excellence
(*aretēs es agōnas*). (DK 82 A8)

Here, once again, *agōn* is joined with *aretē*, this time in the context of a discursive art. Furthermore, in elevating both Gorgias and his art to the best of the arts discovered by mortals, this encomiastic inscription suggests an implicit competition between rhetoric and other contests—athletic, musical, dramatic—for all these would qualify as "contests of excellence." This inscription thus pits rhetoric against other kinds of contests for the title of the art that best prepares one to achieve *aretē:* an *agōn* of *agōnes*.

Concerning the contest between rhetoric and athletics, a comment by Gorgias underscores my point about the importance of the encounter in the *agōn*. In an extant fragment of a speech delivered at the Olympic Games, Gorgias explicitly places athletics and rhetoric next to each other: "A contest (*agōnisma*) such as we have requires double excellence (*dittōn areitōn*): daring (*tolmēs*) and skill (*sophia*). Daring is needed to withstand danger, and skill to understand how to trip the opponent (*pligma*). For surely speech, like the summons at the Olympic Games, calls the willing but crowns the capable" (82 B8). This Gorgianic nugget is packed with commentary on rhetoric's double force of *aretē* and its alignment with athletic *aretē*.

Given the context of his speech—the Olympic festival itself—the metaphor must have resonated powerfully. It seems insufficient, however, to label this a rhetorical flourish and move on. In his explanation of the two kinds of *aretē*, Gorgias uses *pligma*, a noun indicating a particular kind of wrestling move involving a crossing of one's legs with the opponent's, ostensibly with the goal of tripping (hence my translation). At this point what seems like a metaphor becomes something else, as athletic and rhetorical contests become indistinguishable on the level of their requisite riskiness and cleverness, i.e., in the nature and force of *aretē* required. What Gorgias delineates here is a type of contest, one which hails the willing and rewards the one possessing power or ability, *dunamenon,* as exhibited in the *agōn*.

Gorgias' conception of the contest thus called for rhetorical athletes, for a certain kind of cunning and flexibility that enabled rhetors to think on their feet, to anticipate an opponent's moves, and to respond with appropriate moves. In their daring and skill—both required and rewarded—athletics and rhetoric converge as arts of cunning, a concept which will be treated at length in chapter 2.

Rhetoric as *Agōn:* Aeschines' Incorporation of Athletics

Their art infused by agonism derived from and connected with athletics, orators would continue as Olympians of a certain kind, living agonism, questing after *aretē,* and incorporating athletic terminology and situations into their art and speeches. Take, for example, the ongoing *agōn* between the fourth-century orators Aeschines and Demosthenes, and a particular case in which Demosthenes' *aretē* was sharply contested.

The years 341 through 336 were arguably the "heyday" of Demosthenes' rhetorical career. Having provided unfailing leadership during the city's difficulties at the hands of Philip of Macedon, Demosthenes was chosen to deliver the public oration for the war dead at Chaironeia in 337, the utmost honor for a rhetor. And then there were the crowns: a golden crown conferred by the Athenian Assembly signified not absolute rule, but absolute *aretē*. As Aeschines indicates, the crown functions as a material marker of a citizen-leader's virtuosity (*aretē*) and justice (*dikaiosunē*) (Aeschines, *Against Ctesiphon* 10), and when in 337 Demosthenes' friend Ctesiphon proposed that a crown be conferred on Demosthenes for his leadership during the war and recovery, it would have been the third crown Demosthenes had received in five years (Sealey 1993: 201; Demosthenes, *On the Crown* 83). But Aeschines' bitter opposition to Ctesiphon's decree prevented a golden crown from being conferred that year.[8] At stake in Aeschines' charges, as becomes clear in his *Against Ctesiphon* and Demosthenes' famous response, *On the Crown*, is the definition and circulation of *arēte*.[9]

Aeschines' case did not come to trial for six years,[10] and even though the charges failed and Demosthenes received the crown in 330, *Against Ctesiphon* is nonetheless telling for the various ways it uses athletics to situate *aretē* in relation to agonism. The speech therefore illustrates the multiple ways that the bodily concepts of agonism and *aretē* bind rhetoric to athletics.

Against Ctesiphon incorporates athletics in three distinct ways: 1) athletics serves as the well-established milieu for the circulation of honor, and, as such, the athletic contest functions as the epitome of *agōn* and models the ethical production of *arēte;* 2) athletics provides a model by which Aeschines seeks to train his audience to be judicious spectators of Demosthenes' sporting display; and 3) athletics provided a ready taxonomy with which to describe rhetorical performance as agonistic, thus underscoring the first two points.

The three athletic references come late in Aeschines' speech. The first appears in a discussion of *aretē* and tradition, wherein Aeschines argues that the very act of crowning, an official public act commemorating a man's *aretē*, has become cheapened through time: the crowning, he argues, has become more frequent, occurring "out of habit," *ex ethous*, and the proportion of *aretē* is considerably smaller. Athenians, he argues, unlike the judges of athletic contests, are too quick to dole out political *aretē*. In short, the speech takes a typically nostalgic route, as Aeschines argues that contemporary men are inferior to their predecessors, who lived at a time when "honors (*ta kala*) were scarce among us, and the name of virtuosity (*tēs aretēs*) was itself an honor (*timion*)" (3.178).

Aeschines then moves from the appeal to the past to a more contemporary example, a locus where (he argues) old-fashioned *aretē* still exists thanks to the scarcity of its rewards: that locus, of course, is athletic contests. "Do you think," he asks his listeners,

> that any man would ever have been willing to train for the Olympics, or for any of the other crown-bearing contests, the pankration or another of the difficult contests, if the crown were given not to the strongest, best (*kratistō*) man, but to one who has schemed successfully? Not one would have ever been willing. But at this time, I believe, because the prize is rare, and that which is fought for, and honor (*kalon*), and lasting memory from victory, men are willing to risk their bodies, and at the cost of the most severe discipline, surviving the struggle. (3.179–80)

Note how Aeschines invokes Olympic "questing," here characterized as willingness to risk one's body and pay the price of discipline. Furthermore, by setting up athletics as the last bastion of true *aretē,* Aeschines argues that the public crown Ctesiphon has proposed to confer on Demosthenes is already meaningless.

Besides using athletic *aretē* as a way to cheapen political *aretē,* though, in the next lines, Aeschines extends the analogy even further; this time by plugging Demosthenes into the equation as one who is "scheming" for the crown (*diapraxamenō*) rather than one who legitimately deserves it as much as the athletes who have sacrificed their bodies. But he executes this move by placing the audience in the position of judges in a contest of political *aretē:*

> Suppose therefore, that you yourselves are the judges of a contest in political *aretē* (*agōnothetas politikēs aretēs*), and consider too, that if you give prizes to a few worthy men, you will have many competitors for *aretē,* but if you let tribute be paid to those wishing and scheming for it, you will corrupt even reasonable natures. (3.180)

Aeschines thus presents a simple case of crown inflation: the more rare the reward, the more people must—and will—struggle to obtain it. The analogy moves seamlessly from athletic contests to contests of political *aretē,* for both often offer crowns as rewards—clear symbols of virtuosity—and further, both require similar degrees of discipline and training—or at least Aeschines would like for them to. Interestingly, however, since Aeschines here describes a symptomatic yet generalized condition—that of desire and its relation to duplicity—the blame turns on the audience in the Assembly for allowing crowns to be so easily attained—i.e., for allowing themselves to be duped.

In the second athletic reference, Aeschines takes the comparison in a completely different direction. Here, he imagines Demosthenes' rebuttal: that the comparison to athletics is unfair, because contemporary athletes defeat contemporary athletes, and a contest between a contemporary athlete and an athlete from days past is unimaginable, "for [Demosthenes] will say that Philammon the boxer was crowned at Olympia, not because he defeated Glaucus of old times, but because he beat the competitors of his own time" (3.189). He continues by making an important distinction between boxing matches and contests of political *aretē:*

> as if you did not know that for boxers the contest is against one another, but for those who expect to receive a crown, it is against *aretē* itself; since it is for this that they are crowned. (3.189)

In other words, Aeschines avers, the crown is only given when warranted: there is no repeated or regularized competition, and the standard of *aretē* should persist throughout the ages. This is why the audience/citizens need to be trained, he argues, to recognize the standard of *aretē* (much like contemporary judges of figure-skating and diving are expected to know what a "10" looks like, lest they begin doling out "10s" haphazardly). To emphasize this need for the training of citizens, Aeschines again returns to boxing:

> Even, then, as with gymnastic contests you see the boxers struggling against one another for position (*staseōs*), in this manner do you fight him with words all day long for position; and do not let him set his feet outside the bounds of specific charges, but watch him and lie in wait for him as you listen, drive (*eiselaunete*) him to the point of discussion of the lawlessness, and look out for the twists and turns (*ektropas*) of his speech. (206)

Ektropas derives from *ektrepein,* "to turn aside from" or to "avert." The word thus invokes a boxer's deliberate ducking of an opponent's punch, or a wrestler's wriggling form, and Aeschines cautions his listeners to be wary of such quick, wily aversions in Demosthenes' speech.

Aeschines, of course, cannot make the sporting analogy work without an impressive lot of twisting and turning himself. Take for instance the way in which the auditors have become first spectators, then judges, and finally boxers sparring with Demosthenes himself, keeping watch for his cunning moves. The crown, Aeschines implies, is theirs to give; hence, the auditor-voters should become more protective of it, as if they themselves were the reigning champions.

More than that, however, the crossover between the language of athletics and that of rhetoric enables Aeschines to execute these moves more subtly. Take for example his use of the word *stasis*. Here the word for "position" underscores the analogy linking boxing to rhetoric. As a bodily term, *stasis* can be used to indicate a position or posture, and is sometimes used to indicate a boxer's stance, but its meaning moves fairly easily to "the position taken up in litigation"; Aeschines exploits this double entendre to drive home his point about rhetoric's agonism. *Stasis,* as it is commonly known, would later be developed into an entire set of inquiries for forensic rhetoric—inquiries that help determine and establish one's position in a case. It is thus noteworthy that the concept had its beginnings in bodily positions and was frequently used in athletic contexts, as seen in this instance.

By placing the audience inside the "bounds" of the match with Demosthenes, Aeschines accomplishes multiple feats in addition to producing the crowd as protector of the crown: first, he places the audience against Demosthenes, asking them to imagine him as a wily opponent and to thus remain vigilant and watch out for his "twists and turns" (*ektropas*). Second, Aeschines establishes the "illegality charged" as the boxing ring and thus exhorts the auditors to keep Demosthenes within this line of questioning, and not to lose sight of his own (Aeschines') charges (that the circumstances under which Ctesiphon wanted to crown Demosthenes were illegal). Finally, the verb *eiselaunete*—from *eiselausis,* denotes a charge, specifically of chariots. The verb has a pointed force of directed action that suggests guiding, as in rowing, marching, or driving in a particular direction. Here, Aeschines deploys the imperative form of this otherwise bodily/sporting verb to buttress his appeal to the audience to adapt an active, agonistic stance toward Demosthenes' upcoming speech.[11]

Shared Taxonomies

Aeschines' strategy of deploying athletic language, while deft and complex, is not all that novel; the language of rhetoric by his time had a well-established history of borrowing from the language of wrestling, boxing, and chariot racing—and from athletics and athletic training in general. Consider for example, Isocrates' use of *schemata* at *Antidosis* 183, where *schēma* (the singular form) suggests the form or posture of an athlete as well as a figure of speech.

By Aeschines' time, rhetoric and athletics had come to share a peculiar vocabulary, as archaic wrestling terms had wended their way into classical rhetorical taxonomy. Mirhady and Too point to an instance of such a crossover, early in the fifth century, in Aeschylus' *Eumenides,* where the chorus claimed the first of the three "wrestling falls" (*tōn triōn palaismatōn*) in a rhetorical dispute (Mirhady and Too 2000: 240 n. 64; Aeschylus, *Eumenides* 589, 600). Indeed, by the late fourth century, as evidenced by Aeschines' writings, the incorporation of agonistic language in the lawcourts was downright common.

In her book about language and violence in Aristophanes, Daphne O'Regan suggests that it was the older sophists who "seem to have appropriated this metaphor, revised it, and endowed the imagery of martial language with programmatic significance" (1992: 11). Yet while O'Regan is right to credit the sophists with importing agonistic language into rhetoric, I remain wary of this move's status as metaphor. Indeed, as Ruth Padel convincingly argues, the Presocratics did not distinguish between the metaphorical and the literal the way we do today (1992: 9, 33–34). It is important, then, to bear in mind that with such language, a significant transference occurs, in the sense of ancient metaphor: the agonistic language, as Padel puts it, is "not a vehicle for explanation. It *is* the explanation" (34). The movement of agonistic language into rhetoric is just that—a movement, and one for which the older sophists are largely responsible.

The most famous dictum from the sophist Protagoras—"Man is the measure of all things"—appears in a treatise by him that bears an agonistic metaphor in its title, *Kataballontes [Logoi]* (DK B1),[12] where *kataballontes* indicates the act of throwing over, as in wrestling. Protagoras' penchant for "mixing in," *epimeiktos,* noted by Timon (DK A1), likely emerged from his interest in athletics. Protagoras' writings therefore suggest he was interested in athletics as more than a mere metaphor for his discursive wranglings, for in addition to the *Kataballontes* and a treatise entitled *The Art of Debating* (*Technē Eristikōn*), he wrote another one called *On Wrestling* (*Peri Palēs*) (DK 80 A1), wherein he appears to have demonstrated how the art of rhetoric could be of use in the art of wrestling (c.f. Plato, *Sophist* 232d–e).

A locution similar to that used by Protagoras occurs in a fifth-century Hippocratic text, *Nature of Man*. The text begins with a refutation and dismissal of philosophical (read: nonmedical) treatments of the nature of man, a dismissal that culminates in the writer's claim that "such men by their lack of understanding overthrow themselves (*autoi heōtous kataballein*) for the sake of words themselves" (32–34).

Plato, more than anyone else—perhaps because of his own status as a championship wrestler[13]—exploits the taxonomical connection between athletics and rhetoric. In the same vein as the Hippocratic text and the Protagorean treatise, *kataballontes* appears twice in Plato's dialogue *Euthydemus:* first, where Socrates narrates how the title character was about to rhetorically "press [the young Cleinias] for the third fall (*to triton katabalōn*)" when Socrates swooped in to rescue him (277d), and second, where he claims that Euthydemus and his brother Dionysodorus have the problem of knocking down others (*katabalōn*) before falling themselves (288a).

This language, of course, makes sense in a dialogue set in a gymnasium[14] and framed by a description of the brothers Euthydemus and Dionysodorus as

> a pair of pankratiasts . . . most powerful in body and in fight against all—for they are not only well skilled themselves in fighting with arms, but are able to impart that skill for a fee, to another—this is what they do; and further, they are also the best to compete (*agōnisthai*) in the battle of the lawcourts and to teach others how to speak, or to have composed for them speeches such as those in the courts. (271d–72a)

In referring to the pankration, Socrates invokes the violent ancient sport that combined a range of athletic skills—most notably those derived from wrestling and boxing. Still, as the passage goes on to delineate the ways in which the brothers came to excel as pankratiasts—"but now they have put the finishing touch to their skill as pankratiasts . . .

such faculty they have acquired for wielding words as their weapons and confuting any argument" (272b)—it becomes clear that Socrates (in this case) includes rhetoric within the purview of the pankration.

The passage construes the lawcourts as yet another sporting venue in which the brothers excel, hence affirming rhetoric's status as an agonistic event, and—insofar as it is discussed here metaphorically as part of the pankration (the most difficult event)—an arduous one at that. Euthymedus and Dionysodorus are, of course, called sophists, and curiously, where sophists are present in Plato's dialogues, agonistic language abounds.[15]

It seems, then, that O'Regan's claim is on target: the sophists indeed first inhabited rhetoric as an agonistic art. In their work gathering and translating the Presocratic fragments, Diels and Kranz detect this important transformation as well, for they list as a possible imitation of/allusion to Protagoras an instance of *kataballō* in Euripides' *Bacchae* (DK C4; *Bacchae* 199). Perhaps it follows that the free importation of athletic language into rhetoric might be traced to the sophists.

In addition to those terms already discussed (*kataballontes, stasis, schēma*), there are other instances of taxonomical crossover from athletics to rhetoric; one example is *gymnasidion,* a diminutive form of *gymnasion,* which originally signified bodily exercises—the kind of training, as Xenophon has the character Aretē say, accomplished "with work and sweat" (*Memorabilia* 2.1.28)—but which came to also mean rhetorical exercises (Dionysius of Halicarnassus *Rh.* 2.1); *Progymnasmata* later became a common title for rhetoric handbooks, such as that written centuries later by the rhetor Theon.

Still, this discursive cross-pollination occurs most frequently with terms specific to wrestling (e.g., *kataballontes, schēma*). Why wrestling and not, say, javelin throwing? Of all the ancient sports—discus and javelin throwing, chariot racing, boxing, the footrace—wrestling is the sport that for the ancients most exhibited a balance between skill and strength. As Gardiner points out in his early article on the ancient sport, "grace and skill were of far more account than mere strength, and the wrestling matches . . . are but one of the many forms in which the Greeks imaged forth the triumph of civilization over barbarism" (1905: 19–20).

Along these same lines, Pausanias attributes to Theseus the mythico-historical moment when wrestling became a teachable skill or art:

Cercyon is said to have utterly destroyed all those who tried a bout with him except Theseus, who outmatched him mostly by skills (*sophiai*) themselves. For Theseus first invented the art of expert wrestling (*palaistikēn technēn*), and through him afterward was established the teaching of the art. Before him men used in wrestling only size and bodily strength. (1.39.3)

With Theseus, then, wrestling was thought to have moved from a reliance on brute force to a more skillful art that depended on a set of teachable tactics and a clever, responsive body.

By the second century A.D., when Philostratus was cataloguing body types for various sports, wrestling's need for a clever body had solidified. Philostratus emphasizes flexibility of the chest and suppleness of the hips (*Peri Gymnastikēs* 35), and discusses at length the noteworthiness of wrestlers classified as "big little men" (36)—these are men who have an advantage attributable not to bodily mass, but to qualitative differences that make them "lithe, supple, impetuous, nimble, quick, and equable in tension" (36). Such advantages were shared by a compact but wily Odysseus in the wrestling match against the massive Ajax:

> As Ajax heaved him up Odysseus never missed a trick—
> he kicked him behind the knee, clipping the hollow,
> cut his legs from under him, knocked him backward—
> *pinned* as Odysseus flung himself across the chest!
> (*Iliad* 23.806–10; trans. Fagles)

Wrestling is therefore a sport in which the possibility exists for the physically smaller, weaker wrestler to overtake a larger, stronger opponent. As such, wrestling provides the most apt analogue for the sophists' rhetorical art, which is commonly known for its capacity to make the weaker argument stronger (Aristotle, *Rhetoric* 1402a23–26; DK 80 A21).

Furthermore, as a skill-based sport, wrestling had more terminology available for the sophists and others to appropriate in order to produce a "conceptualized rhetoric," to borrow Kennedy's term (1980: 6–10). While wrestling's status as a *technē* makes it the most appropriate sport for sophists to link to rhetoric, it also (excepting the pankration) features the most opportunities for bodily contact, as all body parts are more or less mobilized for the action. As such, wrestling enacted the classic struggle, as wrestlers grappled with legs, arms, heads, skin on skin, muscle on muscle.

Gathering *Clouds*

When the sophists came on the scene in the fifth century, as the story goes, they forced a confrontation between two modes of education— the old, Archaic, and the "new," sophistic. This confrontation, I will suggest, produced not a bifurcation of the two schools, but instead a fusion, resulting in a new figure altogether: a sophist-athlete.

Aristophanes' fifth-century comedy the *Clouds* showcases this very encounter in the form of a dramatic *agōn*. At the center of the *Clouds* is a contest, an *agōn* pitting against each other two arguments (*logoi*) for two styles of education, each of which seeks to cultivate a different type of character. On one side stands the broad-chested, mighty warrior-figure of the old school, *Kreitton Logos* (stronger argument); and on the other, the sharp-tongued, cunning sophist of the new school, *Hetton Logos* (weaker argument).[16] The play also features Socrates as a provider of sophistic training, the shape-shifting cloud-chorus as goddesses of discourse, and one Strepsiades, a comic fool at the heart of the play's action. Strepsiades' name betrays both his character and his quest. The verb *strephō* carries notions of twisting and turning, both in the sense of restless tossing and turning in bed, the state in which Strepsiades appears in the opening scene, and the twisting or turning of a wrestler trying to elude his adversary. Strepsiades the twister seeks out sophistic training, that which he calls *glōttostrophein*, or "tongue wrestling," as a way to slip out of his creditors' "holds" on him.

The two participants in the *agōn*, *Kreitton* and *Hetton*, are generally viewed as caricatures of the old and new schools, binary opposites. *Kreitton* defends his training techniques through nostalgia for the good old days when young boys observed custom (*nomos*) and the civic good by submitting to a particular kind of discipline that emphasized self-control and good repute (lines 962 and 997; O'Regan 1992: 92ff.). The physically punier *Hetton*, however, aligns with the newer sophistic training methods, and is characterized as the proponent of nature (*physis*), set against *nomos* (line 1040). Devoted to immediate results, *Hetton* purports to be able to turn strong arguments against themselves to obtain the immediate advantage.[17]

With the Aristophanic stage quite literally set for a showdown between the two schools, *Kreitton* and *Hetton* prepare to go *mano a mano,* to see which one can win over Strepsiades' son, Pheidippides, as a student. As Daphne O'Regan puts it, "the old-fashioned violence of the hand is pitted against the modern force of the tongue" (1992: 89). Critics generally read the contest and its outcome as indicative of which mode of education Aristophanes favors. But the outcome itself is not so clear. On one hand, at line 1100, *Kreitton* concedes the victory to *Hetton,* suggesting that *Hetton* has taken over Athens' educational system. On the other hand, the ending of the play complicates this easy reading of *Hetton* as victor. When Strepsiades burns down the location for sophistic training (referred to as the Thinkery), the play's ending suggests that *Kreitton* emerges the ultimate victor, and old education (*archē paideia*) prevails. But this reading, like one that crowns *Hetton* the victor, seems too simple given the play's ambivalence regarding outcomes in general (Long 1972: 271 and Kastely 1997a).

In fact, the search for a distinct outcome misses what seems to be the play's major point: it is the *agōn* itself, the encounter between the two schools, and not a "victory" that matters.[18] Here, recall that the *agōn* is more than the one-on-one sparring that is emphasized in most treatments of the topic; recall, too, *agōn*'s original meaning of a "gathering" or "assembly." Similarly, the *agōn* in the *Clouds* depends upon the presence of the audience—the Athenians gathered in the theater, the characters Pheidippides and Strepsiades, and the clouds, which are constituted by the very notion of gathering. As O'Regan points out, "this crowd is invoked at the beginning of the agon; its presence and conduct are vital to the jokes and the argument that conclude it" (1992: 102).

Similarly, Kastely observes that in order to appreciate the comedy of the scene, "the audience must appreciate the value of the agonistic exchanges of rhetoric" (1997a: 34). That is, the *Clouds* does more than point to the contrasts between the old and new modes of education. The drama also offers an occasion to consider the role of the *agōn* in both styles of training; for the *agōn,* in the *Clouds* at least, is what brings the two together, and arguably remains the shared *between*—the very node at which the two training styles converge. It is this point of convergence, this in-between space, that I want to examine more closely.

The *agōn* proper in the *Clouds* is preceded by verbal jousting, exchanges of challenges and threats wherein each promises to smash (*apolō,* lines 892 and 897) the other. The challenges quickly spiral into insults—what might today be called "trash-talking": *Kreitton* calls for a bowl to vomit in because *Hetton*'s very words make him sick (908); *Hetton* calls *Kreitton* a silly old man (*tuphogerōn*); *Kreitton* calls *Hetton* a lecherous man (*katapugōn*) (909–10). They continue:

> *Kreitton:* You're too cocky.
> *Hetton:* And you're absolutely ancient.
> *Kreitton:* You're the one that teaches our youth not to go to school;
>   thanks to you, Athens will soon be comprised of fools.
> *Hetton:* Do you ever wash? (914–18; trans. Dover)

The hearty insult-exchange continues until the cloud-chorus intervenes, tells them to stop battling (*machēs*), and asks them to give their respective accounts of their educational methods (lines 933–38). The clouds' direct intervention marks the beginning of the *agōn* proper.

Kreitton responds by giving a long account of the old style of education, which he claims to be the kind of discipline used to train the men who fought at Marathon (986–87), a discipline that, as O'Regan points out, relies on a set of prohibitions—not to be disgraceful, not to talk out of place, not to seek out loose women; not to commit adultery—precautionary measures that are taken to preserve one's good reputation (*eukleia*) (1992: 93). *Kreitton* ends by admonishing Strepsiades' son Pheidippides to spend his time in the gymnasium in order to obtain a robust, healthy physique as contrasted with the "big-tongued, small-armed" (*glōttan megalēn, pugen mikran*) sophist (1009–18). *Kreitton* thus appeals to the traditional ideals of a strong, lean body suggestive of self-discipline, capable of force.

But *Hetton* appeals to bodily force at the beginning of his speech: "ever since he began his speech I've been bursting to blow it to bits" (1036–38). *Hetton* proceeds to confound (*suntaraxai*) *Kreitton*'s appeals for a constrained lifestyle by privileging the category of pleasure over restraint. In order to do so, he sets himself up as the first to know how "to speak things contrary to the laws and judgments" (*toisin nomois kai tais dikais tananti antilexai*) (1040). *Hetton* then describes a hypothetical situation to Pheidippides wherein Pheidippides is caught in the act of adultery and needs strategies to thwart the angry husband's violent reaction.

If trained in sophistry, *Hetton* argues, the young man will be able to construct an argument on the spot; for example, *Hetton* suggests Pheidippides could appeal to the immortals by citing Zeus' penchant for passion and pleasure over convention. Going along with the situation proposed by *Hetton, Kreitton* asks, "But suppose the man doesn't take any notice? Suppose he starts applying the radish and ashes treatment?" (1086). (Here, as K. J. Dover observes, *Kreitton* is referring to the common punishment of adulterers caught in the act: "a radish was pushed up his anus and his pubic hair was pulled out with the help of hot ash" [1968: 272].) By suggesting that in his own fit of passion, the husband would ignore the appeals to passion, *Kreitton* effectively trumps *Hetton* on his own ground.

These exchanges show subtle shifts and turns in each *logos*'s strategy. Despite the clear polarization between these two *logoi*, at different times each one inhabits the ethos of the other. While *Hetton* invokes violence and military language generally associated with the old school at line 1038, *Kreitton* becomes the clever one in response to *Hetton*'s hypothetical situation. The *agōn*'s end comes when *Hetton* challenges *Kreitton*'s moral high ground by pointing out how the entire Athenian audience is, like *Kreitton,* "wide-assed" (*euruprōktos*) (1083). In other words, it is common for boys in the "old school" to be habitually subjected to anal coitus (Dover 1968: 228)—in short, *Kreitton* and the audience are indeed no different from *Hetton,* who it is assumed finds pleasure in these activities. It is here that *Kreitton* concedes victory by tossing his cloak aside and jumping into the audience. As O'Regan puts it, "In casting off his cloak before deserting to his rival, the *kreitton logos* reveals their fundamental identity when 'naked'" (1992: 98). Thus the two logoi are conjoined, even mixed up; the *agōn* functions to blur the distinctions between the two rather than simply reinscribe them.

One of the upshots of the *Clouds,* then, is the juncture of these two modes of education: their most important shared feature is agonism itself, the use of competition in training. The *Clouds* foregrounds the constant exchange between the athletic, bodily training of the old school and the rhetorical training of the (new) sophists. As I have tried to suggest, it is this very struggle—the twisting and turning inbetweenness of these educational practices—that forms the complicated art of the sophists.

Further, as this book seeks to demonstrate, the emergence of rhetorical training was enfolded with agonistic practices as the *agōn* provided the scene for both discursive and athletic performances, occasions for the enactment of virtuosity. As this analysis suggests, *aretē* was a matter of actions and could only be demonstrated repeatedly (not won). The *agōn,* especially during the time of the sophists, produced a style of rhetorical training based on movement, for the logic of the *agōn* depends on a singular encounter, a necessary response. Sophistic rhetoric, thus fused and infused with dynamics and terminology from athletics, and with old and new techniques, required a particular modality of knowledge production—knowledge held and made by bodies.

Sophistic *Mētis*

An Intelligence of the Body

In his treatise on fishing, the 2nd-century CE writer Oppian offers a lucid description of a dramatic struggle between the octopus and the sea eel:

> There is always fishy war and strife between them, and one fills its belly with the other. The raging sea eel comes out from under a sea-rock and speeds through the swelling sea in pursuit of food. Soon it sees an octopus creeping on the edge of the shore and rushes gladly on a welcome prey. The octopus is not unaware that the sea eel is nearby . . . Speedily she overtakes the octopus and thrusts her blood-red teeth in him. The octopus, of necessity but unwilling, puts up a deadly fight and twines around her limbs, using art, whirling about, now this way, now that, with his tangling whips, by any means throwing its nooses around [the eel], so that he might restrain it. . . . Quickly escaping, the sea eel with its slippery limbs easily slides through the embrace like water. But the octopus twines around the spotted back, around the neck, round the very tail, and then rushes into the orifice of her mouth and the recesses of her jaws.
>
> Even as two men skilled in strong-limbed wrestling too long display their strength against each other; already from the limbs of both pours the warm and abundant sweat and the shifty wiles of their art roam about and their hands undulate about the surface of the body: even so the suckers of the octopus, without order, undulate about, and labor in fruitless wrestling. (*Haleiutica* 2.260–80)

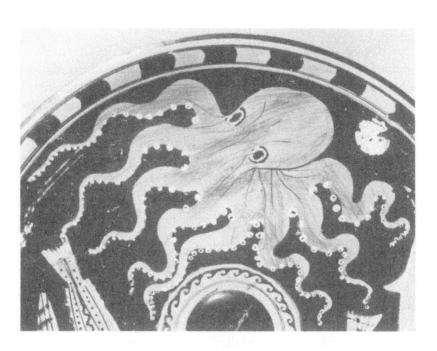

FIGURE 2.1
Detail: octopus on a fish plate: Toledo Museum of Art 77.30.
© The Toledo Museum of Art.

Oppian's vivid account of the sea fight helps illustrate the mode of
agonistic struggle, Protagoras' "mixing in," which, as suggested in the
last chapter, operates in a matrix of response production. The twisting octopus "enfolds" the sea eel with its tentacles, attaching suckers
to its surface, forming a bond between the two, as the sea eel plunges
into the octopus's watery flesh. The struggle produces a fluid mass of
movement, a convergence of forces, which Oppian delineates when
he moves into the wrestling motif: aside from oozing sweat, the "shifty
wiles of their art roam about and their hands undulate about the surface
of the body." Here, art is "mixed in" with bodies, producing a swarming mass of cunning craftiness and flailing limbs. There are elements of
chance, as the sea animals, like wrestlers, grapple wildly without order
(*ou kata kosmon*) (281): the connection to wrestlers here lies mostly in
the quick, furtive movements. Hands undulate; sea creatures' bodies
are thrust in mouths; the movement of bodies parallels, even exhibits,
a roving *technē,* or art.

In subsequent passages, Oppian goes on to detail the role of cunning in the encounter between octopus and sea eel. The kind of craftiness described is a complex mode of intelligence, what the Greeks called *mētis*. The concept of wily cunning, crafty *mētis*, will be the focus of this chapter. As Marcel Detienne and Jean-Pierre Vernant point out in their book-length study of the word, *mētis* generally refers to instantiations of "intelligent ability," all of which emphasize practicality, success, or resourcefulness in a particular sphere (1978: 11).

Oppian's passage therefore demonstrates the importance of *mētis* in struggle, but it also, at the same time, displays the corporeality of *mētis:* the octopus, with its resourceful mass of tentacles, was included in a distinguished group of figures designated as crafty—including, specifically, wily Odysseus, Athena, her mother Metis, and more generally, foxes, wrestlers, and sophists. As this chapter will detail, each figure displays a somatic cunning, and as such, each helps to understand how *mētis* infuses the arts of rhetoric and athletics with a kind of bodily intelligence.

The only extended study of *mētis* is Detienne and Vernant's *Cunning Intelligence* (1978), a protracted diachronic mapping of *mētis*, one which suggests convincingly that the concept itself remained unchanged from Homer to Oppian's time, a span of about ten centuries. Since Detienne and Vernant's study rests on the questions of definition—what is *mētis?*—and location—where is *mētis* important?—their study offers many opportunities for response, extension, and departure. My engagement with Detienne and Vernant will thus elaborate some of their points about *mētis*, most notably the few places where they gesture toward the sophists. At other times, however, my consideration moves beyond Detienne and Vernant's observations, exploring *mētis* as a corporeal category rather than a solely cognitive one—a move the work of Detienne and Vernant supports, but resists nonetheless.

As Detienne and Vernant observe, "there are no treatises on *mētis* as there are treatises on logic, nor are there any philosophical systems based on the principles of wily intelligence" (1978: 3). That there are no ancient treatises on the topic is somewhat unsurprising, given that *mētis*, by its very nature, cannot be apprehended separately from its use. That is, *mētis*, contrary to logic, acknowledges a kind of immanence— it emerges as a part of particular situations, cunning encounters.

As such, *mētis* plays a major role in the *agōn*, as seen in the following passage from the *Iliad*, Nestor's motivational speech to Antilochus before his crucial chariot race:

But, come, my son, put in your heart *mētis*
of every kind, so that the prizes may not elude your grasp.
With *mētis* the woodcutter is far better than by force;
with *mētis*, again, the helmsman on the wine-dark sea
guides his swift ship in the blustering winds;
with *mētis* the charioteer surpasses charioteer.
(*Iliad* 23.313–18)

Mētis is thus the mode of negotiating agonistic forces, the ability to cunningly and effectively maneuver a cutting instrument, a ship, a chariot, a body, on the spot, in the heat of the moment. The force of *mētis* distinguishes action that would otherwise be predictable: charioteer against charioteer, woodcutter who usually relies on bodily strength. While not difficult to detect, this kind of wiliness is impossible to isolate, as the dative form of *mētis* in Nestor's speech suggests the artisans and competitors achieve greatness only with or through *mētis*.

As in the descriptive passage from Oppian with which this chapter began, in Homer's poem there is a yoking of the art at hand to *mētis*. To this end, Detienne and Vernant contend that *mētis* therefore "always appears more or less below the surface, immersed as it were in practical operations which, even when they use it, show no concern to make its nature explicit or to justify its procedures" (1978: 3). Here, despite its reliance on a somewhat questionable surface-depth model of *mētis*, Detienne and Vernant's point remains valid: *mētis* is not an explicit set of precepts but rather a tacit style of movement running through most kinds of action, including thought. According to Detienne and Vernant,

> There is no doubt that *mētis* is a type of intelligence and of thought, a way of knowing; it implies a complex but very coherent body of mental attitudes and intellectual behavior which combine flair, wisdom, forethought, subtlety of mind, deception, resourcefulness, vigilance, opportunism, various skills, and experience acquired over the years. It is applied to situations which are transient, shifting, disconcerting and ambiguous, situations which do not lend themselves to precise measurement, exact calculation or rigorous logic. (1978: 3–4)

What Detienne and Vernant do not explicitly acknowledge, but what their study nonetheless suggests, is the very corporeality of *mētis*. In the passage above, for example, Antilochus is advised to place *mētis* in his heart— *mētin emballeo thumōi*—a bodily locale, the seat of passion or even breath.[1] As described by Detienne and Vernant, *mētis* invokes an idea of intelligence as immanent movement, and as with the example of the octopus and the sea eel, that movement blurs boundaries between bodies and arts as the wiles of art and body converge at the juncture of groping limbs.

Attention to *mētis,* then, makes it difficult to locate *technē*—or thought, for that matter—strictly within the mind or consciousness. In other words, in the *agōn* between the sea eel and the octopus, and in the instance of Antilochus' chariot race, *technē* emerges in a matrix of response, in a series of fluid movements—movements between tentacles, teeth, wheels, horses, all sorts of bodily maneuvering. *Mētis* thus becomes a mingling of quick, responsive impulses. As Janet Atwill suggests in her delineation of *mētis*'s relationship to *technē, mētis* may be contrasted to *nous,* "which is concerned with timeless principles," and may be allied with a kind of philosophical or cognitive *mastery* (1998: 55). As Detienne and Vernant suggest, *mētis* emerges only from shifting or ambiguous situations, thus eluding logical apprehension.

As such, *mētis* becomes a mode of knowledge production, one that informs training practices for athletes and sophists alike. In order to consider *mētis* as the sophist's mode of knowledge production, however, it is important to first explore the cultural production of *mētis* through various Greek figures. From the goddess Metis, to the Homeric hero Odysseus, to the fox and the octopus, figures of wiliness abound in Greek myth and thought. These figural instantiations of *mētis* will help illustrate the various dimensions of the concept, particularly as they emerge in connection with the figure of the sophist-athlete. The chapter will start, then, with the concept's beginning: the story of the goddess Metis.

Metis and Myth

Zeus, as King of the gods,
made Metis his wife first,
and she knew more than all mortals.
But just as she was about to engender the goddess bright-eyed
Athena, then Zeus craftily deceived her
with wily words as bait
put her away in his own belly.
(Hesiod, *Theogony* 886–91)

A marriage, an ingestion, a cerebral birth. Thus is the story of Metis, goddess of cunning, the resourceful one (1. 926). But according to the next few lines of the *Theogony,* Zeus didn't swallow Metis merely to suppress her, even despite his discovery that subsequent to Athena, Metis was to bear a son who would overpower him. Rather, he did so to combine himself with the goddess, so that she could "take counsel with him for things good and evil" (*sumphrassaito thea agathon te kakon te*).

In other words, when he swallowed Metis, a kind of integration occurred: Zeus *became* Metis, offering an early instance of the slogan "you are what you eat." As Detienne and Vernant put it, "[Zeus] is *mētieta,* the Cunning One, the standard gauge and measure of cunning, the god himself become entirely *mētis.*" (1978: 68). At this point, Metis is no longer a singular entity. As a result of the intake, Zeus takes on the cunning and resourcefulness characteristic of Metis, the one who "knew more than all the mortals." The verb *eiduian,* here translated "knew," suggests a mode of knowledge tied to keen perceptiveness, the kind prepared for the uncertain. Metis was thus a goddess equipped with an attunement to contingencies, an inherent preparation for unexpected situations.

The question, then, remains: how did Zeus trick the most keen and perceptive goddess in order to swallow her? Scholars have put forth various arguments on this front, some of which depend on Metis' ability to take on different forms. One version (offered by Goettling [1828: 99] and Paley [1888]) suggests that Zeus convinced Metis to make herself small (*mikran*) and thus more easily consumed. A. B. Cook, however, suggests that what Paley and Goettling gloss as *mikran* is actually *pikran,* possibly a reference to an antidote (*heira pikra*) (Cook 1965: 744 n. 4). Similarly, in commentary on this passage, M. L. West suggests that Metis may have turned into liquid, whereupon Zeus drank her (1966: 403–4).

Whatever particular form she might have assumed, Metis was known as a shapeshifter, as the writings of Apollodorus intimate, for he suggests that Zeus "was united with Metis, who assumed all kinds of forms in her efforts to elude him, and when she became pregnant, he swallowed her, having caught her by surprise" (Apollodorus, *Bibliotheca* 1.3.6). Another key characteristic of the goddess, then, is her ability to morph into a variety of forms, the very ability that ultimately led to her effective "merger" with Zeus.

The goddess Metis thus offers two important and closely related comments on *mētis* as a concept. First, *mētis* is a kind of bodily becoming, insofar as it is transmitted through a blurring of boundaries between bodies, as in the Zeus-Metis exchange. Second, Metis possesses the capacity for bodily disguise; and as the remaining part of this chapter will demonstratre, this status as shapeshifter manifests itself in all figures of *mētis*.

The capacity for disguise is passed along to the most famous product of the Metis-Zeus merger: Athena. Not surprisingly, Athena became the goddess of *mētis*, as the *Homeric Hymn to Athena* suggests, "I begin to sing of Pallas Athena the glorious goddess, bright-eyed, *polumētis*, unbending of heart, pure virgin, savior of cities, courageous, Tritogenia" (l. 29).

Athena's mortal counterpart, at least in Homeric epic, is Odysseus, perhaps best known as the crafty one. Odysseus' *mētis*, of course, becomes apparent during the Trojan War as detailed in the *Iliad;* his most common epithet is *polumētis Odysseus,* Odysseus of many wiles, an epithet that is repeated a remarkable eighty-four times in Homeric epic.[2] In the *Odyssey,* Nestor remembers Odysseus for his *mētis,* as he describes the hero to Telemachus:

> Nine years we wove a web of disaster for those Trojans,
> pressing them hard with every tactic known to man,
> and only after we slaved did Zeus award us victory.
> And no one there could hope to rival Odysseus,
> not for sheer cunning (*mētin*)—
> at every twist of strategy he excelled us all
> (*Odyssey* 3.131–36; trans. Fagles)

Mētis was the source of Odysseus' *aretē* in the *Iliad,* and it assumes no small role in the *Odyssey.* As Pietro Pucci suggests, the notion of return (*nostos*), which is the story of the *Odyssey,* depends on the idea of *mētis* (1987: 17). As such, the *Odyssey*—particularly the cunning, twisting movements of Athena and Odysseus—provides a productive site on which to map this concept of cunning intelligence that assumed such a prominent place in Greek culture, and, as this chapter will ultimately show, in the sophistic enterprise.

Odysseus *Polytropos:* Uncanny Disguise

Despite the fact that it is ostensibly the story of a return, the *Odyssey* reads more like a story of many different turns: a long and twisting voyage, a sequence of encounters, snares threatening to impede movement, obstacles requiring cunning tricks to execute the next "turn." Fortunately, Odysseus—also known by his epithet Odysseus *polytropos,* the man of many turns—is a versatile, flexible hero. As such, he, with the help of his deity-counterpart Athena, has the ability to assume many forms, to take on strategic disguises in order to slip out of the traps set for him along the way. As Pucci observes, disguise functions as a weapon of Odysseus' *mētis* (1987: 85). In the *Odyssey,* then, *mētis* is the most apparent when "Odysseus" is least visible.

Pucci argues further that disguise in the *Odyssey* "is of such an uncanny nature that it is perceived as 'disguise' only when it is detected and exposed—that is, precisely when it no longer functions successfully as a disguise" (1987: 83). It is therefore through dissimulation that the morphology of Odysseus' body helps elicit certain responses from those around him.

In his well-known encounter with the Cyclops in Book 9, Odysseus assumes a discursive disguise of sorts when he introduces himself to the Polyphemus, the curmudgeonly one-eyed creature, as *Outis,* "no one" or "no one in particular." This rhetorical trickery ultimately enables Odysseus and his men to have to take on only Polyphemus, for after Odysseus implements his cunning plan to get Polyphemus drunk on his strong wine and gouge out his eye, and when the other Cyclopes on the island yell into Polyphemus' cave to see who is causing him such agony, Polyphemus' answer translates, *"Nobody,* friends . . . *Nobody's* killing me now by guile (*dolō*) and not by force!" (*Odyssey* 9.453; trans. Fagles). As Odysseus recounts the tale, the other one-eyed creatures "lumbered off, but laughter filled my heart to think how nobody's name—my great cunning stroke (*mētis*)—had duped them one and all" (9.464). According to Odysseus, then, it was the rhetorical trickery of *mētis* that facilitates his and his men's movement out of the cave.

It is on Odysseus' final turn to Ithaca, though, that disguises proliferate most notably. As Douglas J. Stewart (1976: 75) points out, there is confusion on both sides: Odysseus doesn't recognize Ithaca because Athena has cast a dense mist over the land meant to hide Odysseus from the people of Ithaca until he can assume a disguise (13.215ff). But first Athena approaches Odysseus, herself disguised as a shepherd boy who answers Odysseus' queries about his whereabouts. When she tells him that he is in Ithaca, he stifles his jubilance and responds "not with a word of truth—he choked it back, always invoking the *mētis* in his heart" (13.287–88).

Odysseus, wary of revealing his name to anyone in Ithaca before he can assess his household for himself, tells Athena-cum-shepherd boy a string of untruths regarding his status as a fugitive. This moment in the epic provides an instance of *polumētis,* of deified and heroic cunning, as Athena and Odysseus appear to be having a face-off of trickery.[3] Athena interrupts Odysseus' wily tale with laughter, transforming herself into "a woman, beautiful, tall, and skilled at weaving lovely things" (13.325)—yet another, human, disguise. She then praises him for his *mētis,* which, ironically, nevertheless failed to deceive:

> Any man—any god who met you—would have to be
> some champion lying cheat to get past *you*
> for all-round craft and guile (*pantessi doloisi*). You terrible man,
> foxy (*kerdē*), ingenious (*poikelomēta*), never tired of twists and
>   tricks—
> so, not even here, on native soil, would you give up
> those wily tales that warm the cockles of your heart!
> Come, enough of this now. We're both old hands at the arts of
>   intrigue. Here among mortal men
> you're far the best at tactics, spinning yarns,
> and I am famous among the gods for wisdom,
> cunning wiles (*mētis*) too.
> (13.296–99; trans. Fagles)

Athena's chiding speech makes several important points about Odyssean *mētis.* First, she observes the way *mētis* has become Odysseus' mode, his habit, his way of encountering the world. Odysseus' various disguises do not function to "conceal" some hidden "identity," as suggested by Sheila Murnaghan (1987: 14); rather, the disguises *become* his identity, much like the questing of Pindar's athletes (c.f. chapter 1).

Or to put it more bluntly, Odysseus is always becoming something else: in a bizarre twist, his proclamation to Polyphemus that he is no one in particular is actually fairly accurate. What's more, *mētis* becomes both the mode of interaction and the bond between Athena and Odysseus. Athena's speech produces the two as goddess and hero of *mētis,* as partners in craftiness. Most important, however, the brief speech turns on a quick movement from reflecting on *mētis* to crafting the next move, as Athena issues the command "come" (*age*), soon urging Odysseus to consider what to do about his wife's boisterous suitors. In other words, Athena is not all that interested in spending time musing about how wily they are; rather, she wants to put the wiles to work; hence, for both Athena and Odysseus, *mētis* exists only where it is put into practice.

This compressed consideration of Odysseus and Athena elaborates two important features of *mētis*. The first extends the goddess Metis' capacity for disguise. Ultimately, though, Odysseus and Athena turn *mētis* into the capacity for disguise that is not disguise—that is, this very capacity becomes one's identity. Second, *mētis*, by its very nature, needs to be deployed—it does not exist on its own, but only in connection with its use, as seen in the above exchange between Athena and Odysseus. And it is Odysseus himself who provides a conceptual link to two other important figures of *mētis*, the fox and the octopus, to which we will now turn.

Animal Tricksters

The animal instantiations of *mētis* provide figures to be compared with athletes and sophists, the focus of this book. In discussions of athletes and rhetors, comparisons to the fox and the octopus abound. The animals thus provide a critical linking point between mythico-heroic and mortal instantiations of *mētis*. The above-described speech by Athena, for example, invokes both the fox and the octopus, the former directly (*kerde*), the latter tacitly, as will be explained below.

The term *kerdos*, a synonym for *mētis*, suggests cunning trickery, but also yields the root sometimes used for "fox," and as seen in the above passage, Odysseus is often invoked as "the foxy one." The connection between the fox and *mētis* is made also in Oppian's elaboration of the fishing frog's cunning ability to lie motionless in the mud:

> A like device I have heard the cunning fox (*agkulomētis kerdō*) to implement. When she sees a dense flight of birds, having lain down, stretching out her swift limbs, she closes her eyes and shuts her mouth altogether. Seeing her you would suppose her to be in a deep sleep or lying truly dead: so breathless she lies stretched out, deliberating. (*Haleiutica* 2.108–13)

Here, once again, *mētis* is apparent in the ability to assume a deceptive bodily posture—both the fishing frog and the fox can remarkably calm their otherwise alert demeanors to simulate sleep and death. As evidenced by the fact that the fox's name (*kerdō*) also means "wily one" (a crossover that still inheres today with the adjective "foxy"), the fox is no doubt the most commonplace topos of cunning *mētis*.

Just as Oppian uses the fox as a touchstone descriptor for the fishing frog, and Odysseus' character is often elaborated in terms of the beguiling fox, the fox also serves as a comparative figure for athletes and sophists. Oppian's description of the fox in the *Cynegetica* invokes wrestling: "The Fox is not easy to capture by ambush nor by noose nor by net. For she is clever in her cunning to perceive [the hunter]; clever too to cut the rope and to loosen knots and to escape (*olisthēsthai*) from death using shrewd cunning (*pukinoisi doloisin*)" (4.448–51). This description of the fox, packed with words suggestive of cunning and cleverness—*pukinoisi, doloisin, deinē*—enumerates the various ways the fox is capable of escape. The word "escape," *olisthanein*, as Detienne and Vernant point out, invokes an image of the wrestler's oiled body slipping through the opponent's grip (1978: 35). Oppian's fox thus illustrates another feature of *mētis* that will become important later in this discussion: the ability to escape or go elsewhere.

In a reference to *mētis* in *Isthmian* 4, an ode written for Melissos of Thebes, a victor in the pankration, Pindar explicitly connects the fox and the athlete. In this ode, Pindar hopes to "find the favor of the Muses" in order to sing to Melissos,

> For in his heart he resembles the daring
> of loudly roaring beastly lions
> during the struggle, but in cunning (*mētin*) he is a fox
> whirling onto its back (*anapitnamena*) to check the eagle's swoop.
> One must do everything to weaken the enemy. (*Nem.* 4.45–48)

What is noteworthy about Melissos, as Pindar points out, is his size: "For he was not granted the constitution of Orion/ but although he was not much to look at,/ to clash with he was heavy in his strength" (*Nem.* 4.49–51). In other words, Melissos, who was at a physical disadvantage, was known for his knack for finding a way to make himself a stronger force by way of his *mētis* (Gentili 1988: 152).

Here then the reference to the fox—as a figure of *mētis*—articulates a connection between athletes and sophists: the fox, like the sophists, was famous for turning the weaker into the stronger force, creating an advantage out of a perceived disadvantage.[4] Race, in a gloss on this passage, suggests that the act of rolling over and stretching out on its back (*anapitnamena*) could allude to a pankratiast's strategic wrestling maneuver (Loeb edition, 167 n. 3), as the athlete and the animal assume similar bodily positions. *Mētis* thus continues to make itself known through corporeal display.

As we saw in the last chapter, the wrestler and the sophist often find themselves in similar positions whereby the weaker needs to gain some advantage. Similarly with the fox, craftiness helps compensate for lack of size or strength. At times, as in Aesop's fables, the fox emerges as a sophistic figure in the animal world, the sole creature with a crafty tongue. For instance, through clever flattery, the fox coaxes the crow to drop a desirable piece of cheese from its mouth ("The Fox and the Crow" 77). When the ill lion needs food, he calls upon the fox to seek out the stag and "take him captive with your sweet-tongued words" (*logoisi thēreutheisa sois meliglōssois*) ("The Lion, the Fox, and the Beasts"). The fox is a beguiling figure indeed. Just as Odysseus is the figure of *mētis* among men and Athena among deities, the fox is the figure of *mētis* among land animals, exhibiting the capacity for escape and the ability to make the weak strong, whether through cunning appeal or nifty disguise.

If the fox is the *mētis* animal-figure on land, the octopus presides in the sea. Thus, according to Detienne and Vernant:

> Each represents one essential aspect of *mētis* in particular. The fox has a thousand tricks up its sleeve but the culminating point of its *mētis* appears in the way it so to speak reverses itself. In the infinite suppleness of its tentacles the octopus, for its part, symbolizes the unseizability that comes from polymorphy. (1978: 34)

The octopus is the fox's water-inhabiting counterpart; separately, they emphasize different aspects of *mētis,* and together, they provide the most notable models of *mētis* in Greek culture.

Though Oppian gives a glimpse of the *mētis*-endowed octopus in the encounter with the sea eel offered at the beginning of the chapter, a closer consideration will help pinpoint the particular style of cunning the octopus exhibits. Furthermore, as with the fox, the octopus refs back to Odysseus and also to rhetors and athletes. In *Deipnoso-phistai* ("The Learned Banquet"), Athenaeus quotes Pindar's invocation of Ampharaos, who advised his son Amphilochos as follows:

> O son, make your mind most like
> the skin of the rocky sea creature
> in all the cities you visit;
> readily praise the person who is present,
> but think differently (*phronei alloia*) at other times.
> (Pindar frag. 43; trans. Race)

For the ancients, the octopus, here called the "rocky sea creature," was a figure of flexibility; for it was *poikilos,* many-colored, changeable. The octopus's technique, however, differs from that of the fox: while the fox finds a way out, the octopus blends in. In other words, the octopus becomes indistinguishable from the environment, hence the descriptor "rocky."

Pindar was not alone in his invocation of the octopus as a model for this kind of blending in; in fact, a strikingly similar reference to the octopus occurs in the writings of the sixth-century poet Theognis:

> Will, turn towards all friends a many-colored *ēthos,*
> joining with whatever temper each one has.
> Have the temper of the convoluted octopus, which takes on
> the look of the rock it is in converse with;
> now be in accord with this, and then be of a different hue.
> Skillfulness is better than inflexibility (*atropiē*).
> (213–18; trans. Walker 2000a: 139)

Both the Pindaric and Theognidean fragments call on the octopus as a malleable, adaptable figure, a model for action. Jeffrey Walker, in his discussion of the lines from Theognis, points out that "the name *polypous* [the ancient term for 'octopus'], which can also mean 'polyp' in the sense of an amorphous growth, suggests the octopus's power to change not only its color but even its shape, as it passes through narrow crevices and passages in rocks where bonier, stiffer creatures would get stuck" (Walker 2000a: 142).

The octopus, then, a figure of cunning polymorphousness, suggests a modality of response constantly bound up in its flexible, adaptive movement between things—be they rocks, seaweed, or sea eels. This flexibility is directly opposed to what Theognis in the above passage calls inflexibility or *atropiē* (no turns); thus, an appropriate name for such flexibility is *polytropos,* an epithet the octopus shares with Odysseus. Indeed, Eustathius made this hero-animal link most explicitly, when he called Odysseus an octopus (*Commentarii ad Homeri Iliadem et Odysseam* 1318, 36–37).

So these *mētis*-figures exhibit a variety of features. The goddess Metis embodies transformation and disguise; Odysseus and Athena show how this capacity for disguise *is* their identity, thus demonstrating the way *mētis* (not unlike *aretē*) must be performed in order to become apparent. Among animals, the fox specializes in finding ways to escape and in making the weaker stronger and vice versa, while the octopus takes a different approach—blending into the environment through shape-shifting. All these models of *mētis* suggest a modality of response, an affinity for tricks and disguises, a twisting and turning movement, all of which—however differently—return to the body as the place where *mētis* becomes apparent.

Mētis-Hexis

The particular styles of becoming illustrated by these figures of *mētis* thus underscore the corporeality of *mētis:* as a kind of intelligence, *mētis* cannot be thought separate from bodily state. Aristotle quotes Empedocles and Parmenides in the *Metaphysics* to consider a similar point about *mētis:*

> For Empedocles says those changing their bodily condition (*hexin*) deem to change their thought (*phronēsin*): "For *mētis* increases in men according to that which is present." And in another passage he says: "And as they change into a different nature, so it ever comes to them to think differently." And Parmenides also reasons in the same way: "For as each at any time has the mixture of his many-jointed limbs (*meleōn polukamptōn*), so thought comes to men. For each and every man the constitution of his limbs is that very thing which thinks; for thought is that which preponderates." (*Metaphysics* 1009b)

In other words, in Aristotle's view, Empedocles and Parmenides insist on a fusion of bodily and mental states and movements, where different thought trajectories are facilitated by different "bodily conditions," in Aristotelian parlance. The Greek word for bodily condition or bodily state, *hexis,* is indistinguishable from habits and practices (*LSJ*). As M. A. Wright puts it in his gloss on the Empedoclean fragment quoted above, "when men change their *hexis* they change their thinking" (235). For Aristotle, then, Empedocles helps illustrate how disposition is inexorably tied to thought—transformation of one inevitably produces transformation in the other.

The Parmenidean fragment is even more pointed, however, for it gestures to the way in which bodily joints have a range of movement—they are *polukamptēs,* having many curves, or (in music) multiple flourishes. The first sentence in the Parmenidean lines functions more explicitly as an analogy—just as there is a range of movement available in the limbs, so there is in the mind. But with the subsequent line, the analogy dissipates, as Parmenides sutures the limbs directly to thought: "the constitution of his limbs is that very thing which thinks"—thought, therefore, is that which occurs through the limbs and their multidirectional joints: *hexis* equals thought.[5] Thought does not just happen within the body, it happens as the body. In other words, these Presocratics thus held that thought isn't just "embodied"—it is bodily.

Hexis thus describes the bodily "state" that enables particular kinds of cunning, intelligent responses. What happens, though, if one cultivates multiple *hexeis?* The fox and the octopus, for example, have the capacity for changing in response to particular situations—to immediate ecologies. The fox can imitate a dead animal; the octopus a rock; that is, their bodily dispositions change in response to danger. This capacity to change, to assume a new *hexis* (color, morphology, direction, etc.), makes all the difference.

Plato's Cunning *Sophist*

In Book 2 of the *Odyssey,* Telemachus calls an assembly to confront his mother's disrespectful suitors. After several emotional exchanges leading nowhere, and after receiving assurances from Athena (disguised as Mentor), Telemachus resolves to search for his long-missing father. He announces to his nurse:

> I'm sailing off to Sparta, sandy Pylos too,
> for news of my dear father's journey home.
> Perhaps I'll catch some rumor. (*Iliad* 2.396–99; trans. Fagles)

And thus Telemachus sets sail, questing after rumorous news, after some trace of his father's existence and/or whereabouts. Indeed, since Odysseus left for Troy when Telemachus was just a baby, Telemachus can only rely on such indirect discourse, for he does not even know the man for whom he is searching. In fact, when Telemachus finally encounters Odysseus back in Ithaca, Odysseus is disguised as an old beggar, unknown to his son.

Similarly, in Plato's *Sophist,* the Eleatic Stranger and Theatetus set out to find the sophist. Like Telemachus, Theatetus has never seen the object of his search (*Sophist* 239e), and like Telemachus', their search is fraught from the beginning, for the objects of their respective searches elude recognition. As Socrates suggests just before the Stranger and Theatetus begin their quest, sophists, like philosophers, "appear disguised in all sorts of shapes" (*outoi pantoioi phantazomenoi*) (216c).

Both the *Sophist* and the *Odyssey* are thus framed as quests for someone in particular, and both journeys encounter a problem: the object of their search is also always moving to a new place, turning into something else. Hence the searchers can only depend on a kind of rumor, itself constantly morphing.[6]

To be sure, the Stranger and Theatetus initially embark on a kind of "trial" search, a search that leads back to the water. Before setting out in search of the sophist, they will "first practice the method of hunting" (*Sophist* 218d) on the angler. Immediately we encounter the milieux of the *Sophist*—hunting and fishing—milieux that, as Oppian's treatises demonstrate, always depend on *mētis*. As Detienne and Vernant put it, "it is in terms of hunting and fishing that he (Plato) defines the art of the sophist who, in contrast to the philosopher whose wisdom is directed towards the world of ideas, embodies the scheming intelligence of the man of *mētis,* plunged into the world of appearance and of Becoming" (1978: 45). To extend Detienne and Vernant's observation, if *mētis* is concerned with disguise, movement, and a modality of response, then Plato's *Sophist* might be read as a treatise on *mētis,* on a kind of cunning becoming. But first, the angler.

FISHERS OF MEN

The angler should be cunning of spirit and intelligent, since fish devise many and quick-moving devices when they meet with unexpected traps. He should also be quite daring and fearless and temperate and must not love satiety of sleep but must look sharply, wakeful of heart and open-eyed. — Oppian, *Haleiutica* 3.40–45

And so in their attempt to develop a pattern for their sophist-hunt, the Stranger and Theatetus set out to apprehend the angler (*aspalieutēs*). They do so by narrowing down their definition of art to one that fits the angler's. The dialectical movement, which presents a series of decisions based on two choices, beginning with the kind of art, goes as follows: acquisitive art (not productive); coercive (not exchange-based); hunting (not fighting); hunting of the living (not the lifeless); sea hunting (not land hunting); hunting of swimming creatures (not of flying creatures). And then they reach the method peculiar to the angler's sea-hunting (also called fishing), at which point the Stranger and Theatetus oppose that type of hunting carried on by a blow to the kind carried on by means of enclosures. When the angler is placed in the former class, Theatetus proclaims, "I think our search is now ended and we have found the very thing we set before us a while ago as necessary to find" (*Sophist* 221a). Satisfied with their search, the Stranger then proceeds, using the angler-search as a "pattern" (*paradeigma*) for their sophist-hunt.

But as soon as they set out, the Stranger interrupts their new quest, exclaiming that they may have overlooked something all along:

> Stranger: By the Gods! Have I failed to recognize that the man is akin (*suggenē*) to the other man?
> Theatetus: Who to whom?
> Stranger: The angler to the sophist.
> Theatetus: How so?
> Stranger: They both seem clearly to me kinds of hunters.
> (*Sophist* 221d)

And hence they retrace their angler-tracks, pinpointing the place where the angler and the sophist diverge: whereas the angler hunts sea animals, the sophist engages in a hunting of men (*thēran anthrōpōn*) (222c).

But just as the eager Theatetus is about to declare their search successful (*Sophist* 223b), the Stranger suggests that the angler is but one of the sophist's many guises: "for the one we are now seeking partakes of no easy art, but a very many-sided (*poikilēs*) one" (223c). With this observation, the Stranger utters what will quickly become the dialogue's refrain as the Stranger reiterates a little later, "Do you see the very truth of the statement that this creature is many-sided (*poikilon*) and, as the saying is, not to be apprehended with one hand?" (226a). The slippery sophist is thus *poikilos*, in the same way as the cunning, many-colored octopus (*polupous poikilos*) considered earlier. Polymorphousness makes the sophist extremely difficult to catch.

THE SOPHIST'S MANY FACES

Just as the *Odyssey* becomes a story of cunning disguises, so the *Sophist* depicts the sophist as a man of many masks as the Stranger and Theatetus repeatedly try to lay their hands on the masks to pull them off. What they soon realize, however, as we saw with Odysseus, is that the mask does not hide the face, but rather, the mask is the face. It's impossible to unmask an octopus.

The Stranger and Theatetus are themselves cunning shapeshifters, at times, anglers, trying to outsmart the devious, fishy sophist. At other times, in their more motivated moments, the Stranger and Theatetus assume the role of wrestlers: "the saying is right which says it is not easy to escape all the wrestler's grips. So now we must set upon him with redoubled vigor" (*Sophist* 231c). The dialogue is reminiscent of Athena and Odysseus' dueling disguises in the *Odyssey*.

After such erratic shifting, the Stranger avers, the exhausted wrestler-hunters must catch their breath; in the meantime, they will, at the Stranger's coaxing, count "the number of forms in which the sophist has appeared" to them. The forms number six and are as follows: "hunter in search of the young and wealthy" (*Sophist* 231d), knowledge merchant (231d), a knowledge retailer, peddler in production of knowledge (231e), an athlete in the contest of words (231e), and "cleanser of souls" (231e). But the Stranger and Theatetus soon realize that even this extensive list isn't exhaustive; they move through at least two more forms: the juggler and finally the mask or mask-maker: imitator of realities (*mimētēs ōn tōn ontōn*) (235a).

Theatetus and the Stranger thus take another turn, this time to try to delineate the "imitative art" practiced by the sophist. Their first point of inquiry lies in the relation between imitation and reality. On one hand, the Stranger delineates a brand of imitation that uses reality as its guide, "by following the proportions of the model in length, breadth, and depth, and restoring the appropriate colors to each part" (*Sophist* 235d–e). This mimetic art can be distinguished from phantasmagoria, on the other hand, wherein "the artists abandon the truth and give their figures not the actual proportions but those which seem to be beautiful" (236a).

In his discussion of the dialogue, Gilles Deleuze observes that what the Stranger articulates via his phantasm category is the simulacrum (1990: 254), a copy with no relation to an original per se, but which is still a production of the real. John Muckelbauer locates the stakes of the entire search in the copy/simulacrum distinction: "the Sophist, like the Simulacrum, is less a determinate identity than a differential movement" (2001: 242). The multiple trickster–sophist therefore thwarts any kind of search for a unified/identifiable object; what comes to matter in the search is not the sophist's unity or identity but the movement produced by the quest itself.

That the search has been productive is indicated by what they "find" along the way: "Completely separating each thing from all is the utterly final obliteration of all discourse. For our discourse emerges from the interweaving of ideas with one another" (*Sophist* 259e). To "find the sophist," one must follow a network, track rumors. What the *Sophist* displays, much like the *Odyssey*, is a sequence of turns, a carving out of winding paths that produce their own, new encounters. The cunning sophist, like Odysseus, can therefore never be found, only met.

A particularly telling passage connecting the sophist to *mētis* occurs midway through the dialogue when the Stranger says "let us confess that the sophist has cunningly (*panourgōs*) slunk away (*katadeduken*) into an inaccessible place" (*Sophist* 239c). The sophist aligns with the un-trackable fox after he has retreated into a hole—the verb *kataduein* means to sink down or slink into. *Panourgōs*, here used to describe the sophist's style of hiding, is a kind of cunning often attributed to the fox. Aristotle, for instance, in his compendium of animals, offers the fox as an example of an animal that is clever, mischievous, *panourga* (*Historia Animalium* 488b20).

At times, then, the sophist's movement resembles the fox's, darting away into a hole, but at other times, it sounds more like that of the octopus, as when the Stranger observes, "but even now I am not able to see clearly. The man is really wonderful and very difficult to discern, for now, he has cleverly taken refuge in a confounding shape (*aporon eidos*) where it is hard to track him down" (*Sophist* 236d). Much like the polymorphous octopus assuming the shape and color of sea-rocks, the sophist has concealed himself, throwing the hunters off his trail. Similarly, a bit later in the dialogue, the Stranger contends that "the sophist flees into the obscurity of not-being, delivering himself by means of practice (*tribēi*), and is hard to discern in the darkness of the place" (254a). Here, the sophist sounds more like the octopus, jetting off in a trail of ink, released to cover its pursuers in a black haze.

But more important than his likeness to the octopus is the sophist's capacity for making his way through (*prosaptomenos*) the dark, which the Stranger attributes to practice (*tribē*). Alongside its force as "practice," *tribē* invokes an image of a worn path, or, more interestingly, the area where a shoe or a bandage rub, which often produces a blister. In other words, *tribē* names the kind of practice most closely connected to habit and habit-formations and harkens back to Aristotle's invocation of Presocratic bodily knowledge. After much practice, the sophist therefore develops a variegated repertoire of likenesses, of *hexeis,* bodily states that because of their familiarity enable him to move into and out of them with seemingly very little effort. As Aristotle would have it, these states each have their own style of movement, their own directionality, and hence their own mode of thought.

Of course, as in the case with the sophist, such habits and their concomitant capacities for movement against familiar forces, like darkness, for example, emerge from the repeated movement itself: the same movement that confounds the "anglers" seems like second nature to the one who is accustomed to it. Further, the constant repetitive friction between, say, the bandage and the skin, produces something else—in this case a blister. Something else altogether emerges at the juncture between substances.[7]

Theatetus and the Stranger thus have several close encounters with the sophist, mingling with the very attributes of sophistic art: cunning *hexeis* acquired through repeated imitation and careful practice. The Stranger thus observes at the dialogue's close:

> The imitative kind of the insincere part of the art of opinion which is part of the art of contradiction and belongs to the fantastic class of the image-making art (*eidōlopoiikēs*), and is not divine, but human, having been defined in speech as the juggling part of productive activity (*poiēseōs*)—he who declares the sophist to truly be of this stock and blood will, thus it seems, speak the exact truth. (*Sophist* 268d)

Or at least this is the rumor they spread.

The *Sophist,* when read as a treatise on *mētis,* displays the countless forms that *mētis* may take, and, what's more, reveals the futility in trying to capture by means of identification such wily figures as Athena, Odysseus, the fox, the octopus, the wrestler, or the sophist. All these *mētis*-endowed figures have the capacity to take on cunning disguises, and to thereby escape from a seemingly inescapable situation, precisely by acknowledging the *mētis* of *hexis.* For if, in Parmenedian parlance, "the constitution of his limbs is the very thing which thinks," then response, movement, and transformation constitute and are constituted by wily, intelligent bodies.

❊ 3 ❊

Kairotic Bodies

Mētic Kairos

Book 23 of the *Iliad* features a series of contests held among the Greeks in honor of their dead comrade Patroclus. The footrace portion of the games pits three men against each other: "swift Oïlean Ajax, wily Odysseus, and Nestor's son Antilochus, the fastest of all the army's young men" (*Iliad* 23.839–41). As soon as the race begins, Ajax darts quickly into the lead with Odysseus following close behind, his feet landing in Ajax's tracks "before the dust settled" (849). As the crowd screams for Odysseus to win, Odysseus says a silent prayer to Athena, urging her to help his feet. As the two are rushing toward the finish—just in the nick of time—Athena engages in a cunning intervention: she devises a way for Odysseus to win by tripping Ajax even as she makes Odysseus' feet and hands light for victory.

This incident shows Athena deploying her *mētis* with attention to time: had she intervened too soon, Ajax might have recovered for a win; too late, and the race would have been over. In other words, Athena was attuned to the immanent circumstances of the race. This kind of time—time as *timing*—is referred to in ancient Greek as *kairos*.

Forces of *Kairos*

If *mētis* is the mode of the sophist-athlete, then *kairos* is his time. As a number of scholars have pointed out, *kairos*, the ancient conception of time that attends to degrees of propitiousness, does not have a direct English equivalent. Frequently translated as "exact or critical time, season, opportunity," *kairos* marks the quality of time rather than its quantity, which is captured by the other, more familiar Greek word for time—*chronos*. In short, *chronos* measures duration while *kairos* marks force.[1] *Kairos* is thus rhetoric's timing, for the quality, direction, and movement of discursive encounters depend more on the forces at work on and in a particular moment than on their quantifiable length.[2]

Even so, figuring *kairos* as time or "good timing" does not do justice to all the term entails. As John R. Wilson puts it, *kairos* "is a beautifully flexible word" (1980: 177), resonating broadly—spatially, ethically, somatically—and it remains flexible through the fourth century (197). This chapter will revisit the concept of *kairos,* drawing together some of its various valences to show what is at stake in all of them: immanence, movement, and bodies.

In its earliest occurrences, *kairos* functioned—at times directly and at times obliquely—to indicate limits of weight, volume, density, and porousness. In its first appearance in Hesiod's *Works and Days* (694) *kairos* appears alongside advice against overloading a wagon: an overly heavy load will break the axle, delaying delivery and causing the goods to spoil. Hesiod's oraclelike formulation, *kairos d' epi pasin aristos,* "kairos is best in all matters," gives *kairos* what Wilson calls its "ethical-prudential associations" (1980: 179). Such associations can also be found in Theognis, who repeats Hesiod's maxim, and to some degree in Pindar, who sings: "It is best to consider *kairos*" (*Ol.* 13.48). These proverbial sayings encourage attention to what is "right"—the right level of zeal in Theognis' case, and the right amount of praise in Pindar's case. *Kairos* as "due measure," as Wilson describes it, would thus seem to operate in tension with the more opportunistic valences of *kairos* as right time.

As Richard Broxtan Onians argues, however, these meanings become commensurate if considered in terms of the word's more spatialized aspects. In Homer, for example, the *kair-* root is used adjectivally (*kairios*) to indicate a critical, fatal spot on the body, e.g., "where the collarbone parts the neck and the chest" (*Iliad* 8.325), and "on the crown of the head where the first hairs of horses grow on the skull" (8.84). Interestingly, as Onians points out, ancient archers practiced to hit such a spot not by aiming at flat targets, but rather by aiming at "an opening or series of openings" (1951: 345): the fatal spot, that is, is more precisely an opening in the body—a gap or softening in the otherwise protective skeleton, where the arrow can penetrate. It's important to note, too, that such an opening is delimited and formed by the collarbones and the skull, where the bones come together, but not completely—the collarbones, for example, create an opening by not quite meeting each other. This bodily designation thus to a certain degree incorporates the use of *kairos* in the sense of limitation or threshold—as the limited load a wagon can bear in Hesiod's passage.

When figured in terms of archery, a critical, penetrable opening can encompass the spatial, temporal, and ethical all at once: the right place, a "window" of time; the limited amount, "due measure." But Onians goes further, arguing for a heretofore unacknowledged connection to a different word, *kaîros,* one worth considering for the athletic-rhetorical *kairos* I wish to sketch here, for it usefully draws together the forces of *kairos* discussed so far.[3] A key term in the art of weaving, *kaîros* indicates, variously, the place where threads attach to the loom; the act of fastening these threads (*kairoō*); a web so fastened (*kairōma*); and the root was even used to indicate a woman who weaves (*kairōstis* and *kairōstris*). The related *kairoseōn* is used to describe that which is tightly woven.

A line from Pindar, the athletes' poet, hints that the different valences of *kairos* and *kaîros* might be productively kept in play: "If you should speak to the point by combining the strands of many things in few words, less criticism follows from men" (*Pythian* 1.82).[4] The more tightly woven and variegated a piece of discourse, the more "to the point" (*kairon*), the fewer openings or opportunities listeners will have to refute. As this chapter will suggest, the careful weaving together of discourse associated with Pindar's use of *kairos* plays strongly in Gorgias' kairotic style. It is important, then, not to lose sight of the many forces *kairos* bears. While it's difficult to keep in play the various valences of *kairos/kaîros—kairos* as opening, as weaving, as timing, and most notably, as critical, delimited places on the body—this chapter will attempt to do so, as it explores the commonalities found in the various nuances: namely, an emphasis on immanence, movement, and embodiment.

Kairos in Contemporary Rhetorical Theory

Kairos has recently received a good deal of attention in rhetorical studies, and each scholar is invested in one dimension or another. The collection *Rhetoric and Kairos* (Sipiora and Baumlin 2002) chronicles *kai-*

ros's movement into rhetorical theory and reveals the field's focus on the timing and decorum aspects of the concept.

In the 1980s, the late James Kinneavy brought new attention to this previously "neglected" concept by placing special focus on *kairos*'s importance for figuring the rhetorical situation. As such, Kinneavy laid the groundwork for an accommodation model of *kairos*, whereby *kairos* directs the rhetor to consider and adapt to the tones and moods of the situation at hand.[5] *Kairos* as "due measure" or propriety figures prominently in the accommodation model and is supported by Kinneavy's later article, reprinted in the Sipiora and Baumlin collection (2002: 68–73), and by George Kennedy's Aristotelian account of *kairos*. Indeed, Kennedy suggests that this accommodation model of *kairos* is almost wholly attributable to Aristotle when he observes that in Aristotle's version of rhetoric, *kairos* becomes a type of rhetorical *ēthos*, described as "the character of the audience to which the speaker must suit his language and argument" (1980: 92).

Other scholars, however, have viewed *kairos* as a way to reiterate a kind of discursive production, with the rhetor as the creator of *kairos*. Such a version is offered early on by Baumlin, who argues that "the observance of *kairos* becomes above all an interpretation of mutable, contingent, temporal nature, giving the speaker or writer what amounts to creative control over the world he lives in and presents, by words, to others" (1984: 181). Baumlin thus formulates a creation model of *kairos*, one where the rhetor-in-charge creates his or her own openings.

In the early interpretations of *kairos* offered by Kinneavy and Baumlin, *kairos* exists for the most part outside the rhetor, and as such supports a version of rhetoric grounded primarily in rationality and reasoned principles wherein the rhetor/subject analyzes or produces rhetoric as situation/object. Such an art as Kinneavy and Baumlin present, that is, would depend on the rhetor's ability to analyze and act rationally, based on previously conceived notions of what constitutes a rhetorical situation (often recalled in some geometric shape), or grounded in utter confidence in one's own ability to produce *kairos* anew.

Yet while *kairos* re-entered contemporary rhetorical theory in the names of reasoned accommodation and creation, historians of rhetoric have nonetheless presented a different story, making room for the immanent, embodied, mobile, nonrational version of rhetorical *kairos* held by the older sophists Gorgias and Protagoras, as well as the orator Isocrates.

Historical Accounts of *Kairos*

More nuanced historical accounts of *kairos* may be found in Dale Sullivan's "*Kairos* and the Rhetoric of Belief" (1992), John Poulakos' *Sophistical Rhetoric in Classical Greece* (1995), Atwill's *Rhetoric Reclaimed* (1998), and most recently, Scott Consigny's *Gorgias: Sophist and Artist* (2001).

Both Poulakos and Consigny focus on the importance of *kairos* in rhetoric's *agōn* and thereby point to the immanence of *kairos*—the *kairos* of here and now. Consigny's version of agonistic *kairos* is as follows: "*kairos* is an opportunity the rhetor discerns and helps to bring about during the course of the agon, given his perspective and abilities or skills" (2001: 87). Here, Consigny approximates John Poulakos' view that *kairos* is about a kind of immanent awareness. As Poulakos puts it,

> the rhetor who operates mainly with the awareness of *kairos* responds spontaneously to the fleeting situation at hand, speaks on the spur of the moment, and addresses each occasion in its particularity, its singularity, its uniqueness. In this sense, (s)he is both a hunter and maker of unique opportunities, always ready to address improvisationally and confer meaning on new and emerging situations. (1995: 61)

While Poulakos' version of *kairos* is, like Consigny's, tethered to the *agōn*, this connection is nonetheless achieved by a strict adherence to the time and timing dimension of *kairos*. As a result, Poulakos edges toward a kairotic rhetor as temporal genius, an opportunistic "hunter."

While no doubt building on Poulakos' version of *kairos*, Consigny makes a finer distinction in his subsequent explanation of Gorgian *kairos*, tacitly responding to the reason-based creation and accommodation models of *kairos* by taking care to elaborate further the importance of the *agōn*. Specifically, Consigny attends to both the timing and the "opening" force of *kairos* and thus manages to avoid either presenting rhetoric as an art of accommodating a preexisting situation or portraying the rhetor as a creative, improvisational genius. In Consigny's words,

The opening or *kairos* does not exist "on its own," apart from the perceptions and actions of an individual, any more than an opening in a particular moment of play in a game exists independently of the positions and skills of the players. Rather, *kairos* emerges only when a player is engaged in the contingencies of a particular situation and occurs within that situation. (2001: 87–88)

Here, Consigny moves into the language of sport and games in order to crystallize the immanent action of rhetoric. From the point of view of the *agōn*, then, complete creative control or sheer accommodation is rendered impossible. What the *agōn* foregrounds instead is the way rhetoric operates as an immanent art, one in which shifting conditions or countermoves cannot be known in advance. Nevertheless, the immanence presented by both Consigny and Poulakos is articulated primarily in terms of thinking—the verbs "discern" and "address" could easily fall into the category of rational thought. Attending to the embodied aspect of the *agōn*—while perhaps implied by Consigny's and Poulakos' accounts—might broaden immanent "attention" to include different modes of thinking aside from the noetic, diagnostic, rational modes put forth in most accounts of *kairos*.

Janet Atwill's work offers a useful counterbalance in that it enables attention to the embodied aspects of *kairos*. While Consigny figures *kairos* as the moment of agonistic performance, Atwill examines similar issues from the vantage of learning—or the ancients' development of rhetoric as a teachable *technē*. It is precisely the moment when learning is connected to performing that the art's embodied aspects come to the fore. As Atwill observes, "'knowing how' and 'knowing when' are at the heart of *kairos*, distinguishing *technē* from rule-governed activities that are less constrained by temporal conditions" (1998: 59). At stake for Atwill is the kind of knowledge production put forth by the sophists: "knowing when" is difficult to gauge, let alone teach, and it must be achieved through practice.

As with *mētis*, kairotic impulses can therefore be habituated or intuitive—bodily, even—and are not limited to a seat of reason or conscious adherence to a set of precepts.[6] Atwill's treatment of *kairos* in relation to rhetoric tracks through the arts of medicine and navigation, each a bodily art in its own way. Ancient physicians, for example, rely on bodily *kairos*—momentary, embodied perception of somatic symptoms—to make the right diagnosis at the right time (see Lloyd 1970:

362; Atwill 1998: 57).[7] Ship captains both notice and respond physically to changing undulations of the waters. The kairotic arts of medicine and navigation thus help foreground the way *kairos* entails the twin abilities to notice and respond with both mind and body. In other words, the capacity for discerning *kairos*—especially in the context of the struggling *agōn*—depends on a ready, perceptive body.

Dale Sullivan's work on *kairos* and belief supports an account of *kairos* wherein the idea of "discerning *kairos*" (as suggested by both Consigny and Poulakos) can be disarticulated from cognitive recognition as implied by the word "discerning." The result is that *kairos* moves onto a nonrational register—a register that Sullivan argues disappeared when Aristotle made rhetoric into a *technē* (1992: 320).[8] Sullivan regards Gorgianic *kairos* as a "*kairos* of inspiration" (319), and connects it "with romantic concepts of genius and vitalism or with divine madness" (319). Yet if the notion of inspiration is considered somatically as the act of breathing in, or a commingling of momentary elements, kairotic inspiration may be usefully figured in terms of *kairos* as aperture, except this time the opening may not necessarily lie "out there" in circulating discourses or on the body of a foe.[9] Rather, the rhetor opens him or herself up to the immediate situation, allowing for more of an exchange than the creation or accommodation models of *kairos* allow.[10]

Taken together, Poulakos, Consigny, Atwill, and Sullivan offer a version of rhetorical *kairos* as immanent, embodied, and nonrational. In order to further weave together these features of *kairos*, I will now turn to the mythical figure Kairos, who exhibits his own brand of bodily *kairos*. I will then track *kairos* through the art of athletics with its particular immanent, agonal qualities in an attempt to elaborate the role bodies play in "discerning" *kairos*. Doing so maintains a variegated account of *kairos*, one that draws out the contributions of Consigny, Poulakos, Atwill, and Sullivan by tuning in to dynamics, movements, words, rhythms, and bodies. After elaborating a bodily version of *kairos* in athletics, the chapter will end by considering Gorgias and the particular ways his art is shot through with bodily *kairos*.

The Instructive Body of Kairos

Kairos first appears as a mythical figure in the middle of the fifth century BCE, when Ion of Chios dedicates a hymn to him (Cook 1965: 859; Pausanius 5.14.9). It was Lysippos, we are told, who in the later

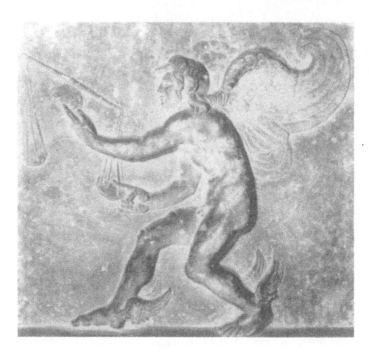

FIGURE 3.1
Marble relief depicting Kairos.
© Turin Museum, Italy.

part of the fourth century BCE, "enrolled Kairos among the gods" (Himerius 14.1) by rendering him visible in the form of a body. The bronze Lysippean statue is no longer extant, but copies, such as the marble relief pictured in figure 3.1, bear witness to the spirit and energy of Lysippos' work.

Exhibiting the bodily form of an athlete, Kairos is depicted as a well-muscled winged figure perched on a stick, balancing a set of scales on a razor blade. The muscles are tense, the gaze forward, wings spread, back foot raised slightly, ready to change direction. His three sets of spread wings suggest he may already be in motion.[11]

That Kairos was sculpted by Lysippos, who was best known as a sculptor of athletes, has not yet been considered in rhetorical scholarship. For classical scholars, however, the sculptor's relation to Kairos has presented something of a quandary. A. B. Cook, for example, puzzles over the significance of Kairos's sculptor. The idea that Lysippos would render "such a curious piece of allegory," Cook argues, is "a problem which has never been squarely faced" (1965: 859). Instead of addressing the problem himself, Cook goes on to speculate that the statue is not allegorical at all, but rather another way for Lysippos to render a graceful male form. More recently, classical archaeologist Andrew Stewart argues (1978) that the statue of Kairos functions as an instructional message about Lysippos' own art of sculpting, thus more-or-less skipping over the question of Kairos's relation to Lysippos' other athlete-subjects.

But textual evidence suggests that Kairos's connection to athletics goes much further than graceful male forms, or self-reflexive meditations on sculpture. Indeed, as Pausanias points out, the entrance to the stadium at Olympia was flanked by two altars, one in honor of Hermes, god of the Contest (*Hermou . . . Enagōniou*); the other devoted to Kairos and marked by Lysippos' statue (5.14.9). Hence ancient athletes, upon entering the stadium, were invited to observe Kairos's role in the *agōn:* the statue no doubt bears the significance of *kairos* to the athlete's art, the immanence of competition with its ever-shifting conditions, and the necessity of remaining open and responsive to such changes.

If Lysippos gave Kairos a body, the poet Posidippos gave him a voice, composing an epigram for the statue's base in the third century BCE:

—Where is your sculptor?—Sikyon.
—What is his name?—Lysippos.
—Who are you?—Kairos, subduer of all.
—Why do you stand on tiptoe?—I run quickly.
—And why do have wings on both your feet?—I am swift as wind.
—Why do you hold a razor in your right hand?—As proof to men that I am sharper than any sharp end.
—Why does your hair grow over your face?—For one who encounters me to grasp.
—God! Why does it become bald behind?
—For once my winged feet pass by, even if desiring to, no one can grasp me from behind.
—For what reason did the artist fashion you?—For your sake, stranger, and he placed me before the entrance as a lesson. (*Anth.Pal.* 16.275.7)

This epigram gives Kairos the epithet *ho pandamatōr,* a term that may be translated "subduer of all." The root verb *damaō, damazo* can mean subdue or tame in the sense of "conquer" or "gain mastery over," and is sometimes used, as in Pindar's *Pythian* 8.80, in the context of athletics as a synonym for winning. Visually, the epithet inheres in the god's accoutrements; for Cook notes that the razor, scales, and wings connect Kairos to Nike and Nemesis, goddesses of victory and overcoming (1965: 860–61). The epithet's relation to Kairos seems straightforward: Kairos presses upon all—from wagons, poems, and songs, as seen with Hesiod, Theognis, and Pindar, to contests, arts, and bodies.

In addition to ascribing ubiquitous force to Kairos, the Posidippean epigram mentions Kairos's capacity for movement no less than three times (lines 4, 5, and 9): by referring to his ready stance (on tiptoe); mentioning his swiftness; and comparing him to wind. With his winged feet and ready stance, Kairos will blow by mortals, who, if they themselves are not ready to seize him in advance, will be left swiping at his bald pate.

This epigrammatic obsession with Kairos's movement, if taken alongside Stewart's reading of the statue, is right in line with Lysippos' own obsession. As Stewart points out, this statue was unlike Lysippos' others in that it was not commissioned, but rather a statue made by the sculptor for the sake of his art. As such, Stewart reads the statue as Lysippos' manifesto, a demonstration of his ability to render the most challenging aspects of sculpting human bodies—those of symmetry and movement (1978: 171). Lysippos thus casts the two in perfect balance— kairotically.

Taken further, Lysippos' manifesto in bronze may also be read as a commentary on his art's convergence with the art of his subjects—it was, after all, athletes to whom the Greeks attributed bodily virtues of symmetry and movement, and their capacity for balancing the two is developed over time, through practice, and placed on display in every performance. Lysippos, by virtue of his commissions to sculpt athletes, repeatedly tried to cast them in motion, thereby gaining an intimate familiarity with the importance of *kairos* for athletics as well as for his own art.

Grappling most directly with this question of the statue's *raison d'être*, however, is the inscription's final line. While the rest of the epigram is devoted to interpreting Kairos's various physical features, most of which remind the onlookers of his swiftness and movement, the final line raises the perplexing question, and the very one sidetracked by Cook: why would a sculptor of athletes give you, Kairos, a body? The answer itself is brief and fleeting: Lysippos crafted Kairos for the sake of the statue's beholders, as a lesson, a *didaskalia*.[12]

Stewart's suggestion that the "lesson" is confined to sculpting omits the important factor of location. Put simply, if the lesson was for sculptors, why would the Lysippean Kairos be placed at the entrance of the stadium at Olympia? The strong possibility remains that Lysippos' statue was dedicated to his subjects as much as to himself: the statue, that is, stood as a testament to athletes' bodily symmetry and motion even as it displayed Lysippos' ability to render these features in bronze. Moreover, the statue stands as a visible reminder of the conditions inside the stadium, the necessity of attending to the immanent, embodied, circumstance of competition. The value of athletic bodily *aretē* and the importance of embodied thought-in-motion combine in Lysippos' statue to underscore the importance of *kairos*—in all its variegated resonances—for athletics.

Supporting this reading and (most likely) the statue itself is a base found at Olympia carved in the form of a large astragal, a knucklebone (Kurke 1999: 293; Stewart 1978: 163 n. 2). The bones of sheep and goats, knucklebones were used like jacks in children's games, and bore strong connections to fate and sacrifice (Kurke 1999: 288). Though the statue base's association with Kairos is contested, Stewart, Kurke, and Guarducci (1966: 291–92) argue that the link is there, and Kurke goes on to use the assumed association to link *kairos*—through the astragal— with the three Graces. According to Kurke, "Grace (*charis*) was the highest virtue of aristocratic style, denoting the perfection of bodily form and movement" (292). Kurke's point is underscored too by the graceful form of Lysippean Kairos, his Posidippean epigram, and the movement reiterated in both. The possible connection to *astragoloi* nonetheless remains intriguing, for as Kurke points out, *astragoloi* bore an intense bodily association since they derived from the bodies of animals (288)—this connection to bodies, notably bodies of sacrificial animals, according to Kurke, "endows them with fateful power" (290). For Kurke, the statue and its base combine the luck of the knucklebone throw with what Kurke calls "that other cardinal virtue of aristocratic embodiment—*kairos*, the opportune moment and the instinct to seize it in a contest" (293). It is worth noting too that in the context of athletics, for Kurke at least, *kairos* becomes figured as instinctual, a bodily capacity for instantaneous response.

The Lysippean statue thus helps figure *kairos* as a bodily virtue of movement and instinct. When Lysippos' rendition of Kairos is reconnected to the embodiment of timing and the *agōn,* as suggested by its location at Olympia, *kairos* becomes attuned to the rhythms and movements of all forces in the *agōn*—stops and starts, lunges and hedges, trips and falls, and the opportunities therein. Lysippos' statue, then, stands as a reminder that kairotic inspiration may be figured as a receptive, open, body—a body, like the god Kairos, casting a broad gaze, exhibiting an intense yet open stance, a body that radiates readiness.

In the context of athletic games, then, time becomes enfolded with bodies, and as the wings on Kairos's feet and back suggest, those bodies, like time itself, are always on the move. Kairotic athletes must therefore constantly invent and combine—in the sense of the *kaīros* from weaving—moves in the *agōn,* on the spot, in the blink of an eye, or in the split-second movement of a limb. It is worth noting that Kairos gained a toehold on divinity in the fifth century and was given a body by a sculptor of athletes in the fourth century—exactly the timespan in which rhetoric and athletics came together most pointedly. Such a convergence fits nicely with the sophist Protagoras' effectiveness in drawing together rhetoric and the *agōn,* even as he became the first to "expound on the power of *kairos*" (DK 80 A1 52).

Sophistic *Kairos*

In the realm of sophistic rhetoric, *kairos* emerges as a kind of immanent, rhythmic, embodied practice. The sophist Gorgias hit on this kind of agonistic immanence when he took the stage in the theater at Athens and challenged the audience to "suggest a subject," a move which, according to Diogenes Laertius, showed that he "would trust to the moment (*tōi kairōi*) to speak on any subject" (A1a). In other words, Gorgias would submit to immanence in a particular rhetorical moment—a *kairos*—for movement, to take discourse somewhere else. So much has been made of Gorgias' kairotic art that it seems the book should be closed on the topic. *Kairos,* after all, is widely noted as that which distinguishes the sophistic art.[13]

Elaborating *kairos* as a major principle of sophistic rhetoric, John Poulakos writes that the concept realizes "that speech exists in time and is uttered both as a spontaneous formulation of and a barely constituted response to a new situation unfolding in the immediate present" (1995: 61). Such an understanding of *kairos,* as this chapter has heretofore suggested, is, in the words of James Kastely, "fluid and provisional" (1997b: 224). In other words, to paraphrase Eric White, *kairos* necessitates that thought always be on the move in order to resist "freezing" (1987: 41).

In his defense of Helen, a speech in which he interrogates the prevailing assumptions about Helen's responsibility for the Trojan War, Gorgias demonstrates this sense of the term by drawing the audience in through his mobile discourse. When Gorgias suggests that the power (*dunamis*) of speech could be the reason for Helen's flight to Troy, he also performs his point, as Gorgias and his listeners become implicated in his own speech. In other words, just as Helen was carried off to Troy, Gorgias' listeners will be moved away from their convictions regarding Helen's culpability.

He begins this line of argument by calling speech a "great ruler" (*dunastēs megas*) that can effectively "stop fear and relieve pain (*lupēn*) and instill joy and increase compassion" (*Helen* 8). Before he goes on to develop this point, Gorgias addresses his hearers in the imperative: "listen (*phere*) as I turn (*metastō*) from one argument (*logon*) to another" (9). The verb *metastō,* from *methistēmi,* here translated as "turn," is a verb of movement. It generally takes the force of "to transform" or "change," as in to change form or position.

This moment of direct address thus marks a critical—and literal—turning point in the *Helen:* not only does it flag a transition from one argument to the next, but it signals the transformation of Gorgias himself in that discursive movement. He becomes a wing-footed rhetor, noting openings in the arguments concerning Helen to take them (the audience *and* the arguments) somewhere else, namely to a place where Helen is free from blame. Gorgias does more than catalogue arguments, he cultivates an ethos that morphs between *logoi.*

It is therefore the *turn* itself, not the *logoi,* the very act of being taken elsewhere that Gorgias foregrounds and mimics when he directs those present to listen, *phere. Phere* comes from the verb *pherō,* which means "to bear" or "to carry" but can also (at the same time) indicate a yielding or producing, as a cow producing (and hence bearing) milk. The act of listening, then, becomes just that: a productive, active, transformative act for hearers and speakers. At this point, Gorgias orders his listeners to bear and produce his act of turning. This moment of direct address, then, emphasizes the transformative encounter produced through discourse. Gorgias is demonstrating what might have happened to Helen's body by showing the *dunamis* of his art.

Gorgias' speech thus inscribes him as a *mētic* shapeshifter—for the sake of "argument"—inserting Gorgias himself into the situation at that particular moment, imploring those present to *phere,* to bear and produce the transformative rhetorical encounter: "Listen as I turn."

Bringing the movement of *kairos* to bear on Gorgias' own rhetorical practice reveals the limitations of the "accommodation" and "creation" models of *kairos* discussed earlier. While these versions of *kairos* require the "rhetor"—a discrete, rational being—to decode a "rhetorical situation" from outside (step one), and then consciously select or create "appropriate" arguments (step two), *kairos* provides a point of departure from reasoned, linear steps—even from consciousness. As Eric White puts it, "The rhetorical practice of the sophist who allows *kairos* to figure in the invention of speech will issue, then, in an endlessly proliferating style deployed according to no overarching principle or rational design. The orator who invents on the basis of *kairos* must in fact always go beyond the bounds of the 'rational'" (1987: 21). White raises an important point about *kairos*'s relationship to reason: the fleeting movement of *kairos* necessitates a move away from a privileging of "design" or preformulated principles. At times, however, these so-called principles could be so habituated as to not require "thinking" per se. They depend instead largely on the rhetorical encounter itself and the *kairos* pressing on—subduing—the encounter.

Rather than just insisting that Gorgias' version of *kairos* moves rhetoric beyond reason, I want to consider how the body figures prominently in this movement. In order to do so, it will be useful to read Gorgias' mobile theories of kairotic discourse alongside his theories of the body.

In Plato's *Meno,* Gorgias is said to have followed his teacher Empedocles in his belief that "existing things have some effluences (*aporroai*) . . . and pores into which and through which the effluences are carried" (76C). This theory of extramission, which will also be discussed more generally in chapter 7, held that effluences, fluids, films, or smells emitted, transmitted through the body were suited to sensory perceptions. Pores were thus thought to operate as tiny channels, moving various transformative substances—such as air or passion—through the body. Gorgias was said to have thought that fire moved through pores of materials in a similar manner, as evidenced in Theophrastus' refutation of Gorgias' theory that combustion from mirrors and other shiny surfaces takes place "'by means of the fire passing away through the pores'" (DK 82 B5).

For Gorgias, bodies and souls, like bronze and silver, were porous entities that allowed effluents and other substances (words, fire) to pass through. In this Gorgias agreed with the Hippocratics, who also followed Empedocles, and who, according to Padel, originated the "western medical portraiture of the infinitely penetrable body" (1992: 58).

Recalling the *kairios* of Homer's warriors, the porous body of Empedocles offers a microscopic version of the body's skeletal gaps where arrows can pass through to the life within. The movement of the arrow can thus be viewed as analogous to the movement of fire in Gorgias' theory of combustion. Given the sophistic penchant for relating rhetoric to other arts and sciences, it makes sense that Gorgias' figuring of kairotic bodies in the realms of perception and combustion transfers easily into the realm of discourse. Perhaps it is no coincidence that the sophist's speeches were sometimes referred to as "torches" (Smith 1921: 359).

Gorgias' theory of the effluence-pore relation shapes his version of rhetoric in a number of ways, allowing us to consider more specifically how *kairos* figures into his rhetoric. The famous *pharmakon* passage from Gorgias' *Helen* brings together his theory of discourse with his theories of the porous body:

> The power of speech has the same relation to the disposition of the soul as the application of drugs on the disposition of the body. For just as different drugs draw different juices out of the body, and some end disease but others end life, so also some speeches produce pain, some enjoyment, some fear; some instill courage in hearers; some drug and beguile the soul with a kind of evil persuasion. (*Helen* 14)

For Gorgias, *logos* can move through the *psyche* like drugs through the body's interior passages. Speech's effects, that is, can be as potent as hemlock. Here Gorgias focuses on the different orders of change that may be elicited or produced through drugs and discourse. While the passage begins with a clear-cut analogy, however, it ends with a list of descriptors for speech that can be just as easily applied to psychotropic drugs, which were widely known to produce pain, enjoyment, fear, and courage. This slippage combines with Gorgias' use of "drug" (*pharmakeusan*) as the passage's final verb with speech as the implied subject—"some drug and beguile the soul"—to suggest the metaphor's dissipation: *logos* becomes a type of *pharmakon*.

Jacques Derrida has written a good deal on the Greek word *pharmakon* and its relationship to writing. In his reading of the concept through several Platonic dialogues, Derrida points out that "the *pharmakon* is that which, always springing up from without, acting like the outside itself, will never have any definable virtue of its own" (Derrida 1981: 102). That is, a *pharmakon* (translated variously, as Derrida points out, as "drug," "remedy," "poison") can only be considered in relation to something else, some other body, and its effects on a particular body cannot be known in advance. As Derrida puts it, "in order for this *pharmakon* to show itself, with use, to be injurious, its effectiveness, its power, its *dunamis* must, of course, be ambiguous" (103).

Derrida may well be referring to Gorgias' assertion of the *dunamis* of *logos* toward the beginning of the *Helen:* "Speech is a great ruler (*logos dunastēs megas estin*) that with the smallest and most invisible body (*hōs smikrotatōi kai aphanestatōi*) accomplishes most godlike works. For it is strong enough (*dunatai*) to stop fear and to relieve pain (*lupēn*) and to instill joy and to increase compassion" (*Helen* 8). Here, the *dunamis* of *logos*—its potency—acts on and through the body. The verb here translated as "to instill," *energasasthai*, involves making or producing something in something else—in this case, joy in the listeners. The word for pain, *lupē*, often designates pain of the body. Furthermore, just as a drug is a substance with its own kind of body, so speech, for Gorgias, doesn't merely operate on bodies, but, as Gorgias hints here, discourse itself operates as a body, albeit difficult to discern separately from its effects.

Taken together, these two critical passages in Gorgias' speech link the art of discourse with Gorgias' Empedoclean theory of effluences. First, the speech-as-*pharmakon* requires a porous body to pass through in order to incite pleasure or courage, or to induce pain or fear. Second, however, *logos* itself bears a body—the smallest and most invisible body (*hōs smikrotatōi sōmati kai aphanestatōi*)—a body that both moves and mingles with the body/soul it effectively drugs.

Gorgias emphasizes the importance of speech's movement into and out of bodies in his discussion of songs and incantations at 10: "Songs inspired through words are the bearers of pleasure and the banishers of pain." The words translated here (and by Kennedy) as bearers and banishers—*epagōgoi* and *apagōgoi*—are a set of antithetical terms with the same root, *agō*—to lead. Here, Gorgias uses songs to parallel instances of speeches that transport certain sensations—e.g., pleasure and pain—in and out of the body.

Just as in the instance of drugs, for Gorgias, music does not serve merely as an analogue for speech, but is a critical force in discourse-production as well, as he emphasized the rhythmic movements of discourse. One of Gorgias' legacies, as it is widely thought, is the introduction of rhythm and poetic style to the art of words. As Diodorus Siculus points out, "(Gorgias) was the first to use extravagant figures of speech marked by deliberate art: antithesis and clauses of exactly or approximately equal length and rhythm and others" (DK 82 A4). Similarly, Suidas contends that Gorgias "was the first to give the rhetorical genre the verbal power and art of deliberate culture and employed tropes and metaphors and figurative language and hypallage and catachresis and hyperbaton and doublings of words and repetitions and apostrophes and clauses of equal length" (DK 82 A2).

Gorgias thus blurred the distinctions between lyrical poetry and rhetoric. As Charles P. Segal notes, "Gorgias, in fact, transfers the emotive devices and effects of poetry to his own prose, and in doing so he brings within the competence of the rhetor the power to move the *psyche* by those suprarational forces which Damon is said to have discerned in the rhythm and harmony of the formal structures of music" (1972: 127). Specifically, Damon studied music's effects on the movement (*kinesis*) of the *psyche* (Segal 1972: n. 103). Bromley Smith compares Gorgias' speech to "a symphony[,] because when read aloud it recalls a piece of music; for it has the cadences, tonal effects, diminuendos and crescendos of a sonata" (1921: 350), and Edward Schiappa argues that a proper title for Gorgias is "prose rhapsode" (1991: 245), thus marking Gorgias' "striking and almost musical" style (1991: 251) and his hybridized (poetic-prosaic) discursive strategies. In his remarkable study of euphony and the Greek language, W. B. Stanford notes that Gorgias "showed how elaborately and effectively a prose-speaker could use effects of rhythm and assonance to influence his audience" (1967: 9). Gorgias is thus the most musical of the sophists.

In arguing convincingly that rhetoric and music were sister arts (1967: 27), Stanford usefully details the shared features of speech and music, thus helping enumerate the ways in which Gorgias attended to musicality. For Stanford, the kinship between speech and music lies in acoustic effect and may be divided into five subcategories: pitch, tone, tempo, intensity, and rhythm.[14] Material, bodily sound was one of the few ways ancient orators could produce something like special effects — from the startling boom produced by a deep-toned shout (which Stanford calls intensity) to the melodic smooth-textured rhythms of assonant discourse. Gorgias famously drew from all the available means of euphony as he yoked poetics and rhetoric.

In his study of rhetoric's relation to poetics, Jeffrey Walker (2000a) offers Gorgias' Funeral Oration fragment as an instance of hybridized prosodic poetry, observing that it employs "oppositions, symmetries, balances, repetitions, echoes, and rhythmic phrasings" (2000a: 23). Gorgias simultaneously conjoined the rhythmic quality of language brought out by careful prose composition with the physical effects allowed by vocal manipulation — attention to pitch, tone, and tempo. Attuned to the effects of variation, melodies, and tones in speech, Gorgias and his physical voice thus become a critical part of the discourse, as the harmonies of poetry meld with the art of speaking. The net effect is an art that attends to tempo, the formation of rhythm through stops and starts, pauses and gaps, and the tightly woven paratactic style discussed at length by Jarratt (1991: 22–25).

Most of the figures Gorgias is credited with having brought to the domain of rhetoric suggest some sort of movement. For example, tropes (*tropais*), from *tropē*, meaning turn, turning, and *tropos* can be used to indicate musical harmony, or a particular mode. Metaphor, from *metaphora,* transport, haulage, change, even a passing phase of the moon, was itself "transferred" to indicate the "transference of a word to a new sense." Hypallage (*hypallagē*), a term for interchange or exchange, such as the exchange of women, or the change of regime or the color of wine (*LSJ*), came also to denote a verbal play on shifts in shades of meaning; apostrophe from *apostrephein,* a turning away, a bend in the stream, or, in rhetoric, a turning away from others to address one (*LSJ* 220).[15]

Most of these figures are verbs made into nouns, and most mark the twists and turns (and potential twists and turns) that discourse can produce. The figures Gorgias used in discourse production are therefore tools of movement, facilitating the kind of discursive action that was later dubbed "to Gorgianize" (DK 82 A35). The cumulative effect of these Gorgianic tropes and figures is summed up nicely by George Kennedy: "On Gorgias' lips oratory became a tintinnabulation of rhyming words and echoing rhythms" (1980: 29). In other words, sophistic rhetoric could be said to have its own score.

Chapters 5 and 6 will discuss the bodily aspect of music for the ancients; how, for example, music was thought to "move in" to the soul through the body, and to reproduce its own dispositions. Such a notion seems to inhere, too, in Gorgias' own incantations. Together with his notion of speech-as-*pharmakon,* Gorgias' theory of speech-as-music suggests that the kairotic body is foremost on his list of rhetorical considerations—speech itself becomes a mobile body, shot through with *kairos.*

Gorgias' somatic version of *logos* further underscores a doubly kairotic tenor of his rhetoric in that it reintroduces the spatial origins and mobile features of *kairos*—the *kairos* that depends on openings as much as it depends on movements, a mingling of porous, effective bodies. A bidirectional *kairos* becomes clear as the wing-footed rhetor speeds through kairotic openings. A *pharmakon*-style *kairos,* moreover, marks a particular quality of discourse, one that doesn't necessarily pass through the mind to obtain meaning, but rather operates at the level of the body, on the level of effect or sensation—inciting pain or pleasure.[16]

The production of a bodily state, be it the emission of particular fluids, the relief of pain, or the "leading in" of pleasure, depends on the singular encounter between song and body, drug and body, word and body. Such relational specificity helps account for the importance of *kairos* in sophistical rhetoric, as well as for the general dissatisfaction with Gorgias' attempts to write about *kairos.* Dionysius of Halicarnassus, for example, complains that Gorgias did an unsatisfactory job of writing about *kairos:* "No orator or philosopher has up to this time defined the art of the 'timely,' not even Gorgias of Leontini, who first tried to write about it, nor did he write anything worth mentioning" (DK 82 B13). Untersteiner contends, however, that Dionysius only considered "pedantic formal classifications" to be worth mentioning (Untersteiner 1954: 203 n. 11).

Enumerating "precepts" of *kairos* would prove counter to Gorgias' rhetoric, and to *kairos* itself. It is precisely because of this relational specificity that Gorgias cannot offer a manual of *kairos*—or at least not one that would satisfy Dionysius. Perhaps the *Helen* could be seen as such a manual, however, with its comparison of speech to drugs and witchcraft, both of which are intensely circumstantial and bodily. The speech, that is, offers a performative demonstration of the way *kairos* folded so neatly into bodies in motion; as such this just might be the only form such a manual can take.

Such a manual flickers on the scene much later in a treatise on sport entitled *Peri Gymnastikēs* (*On Gymnastics*) by the sophist Philostra-tus. Here the author hits on a kind of kairotic training when detailing the work of the wrestling teachers (*paidotribai*): "How many different kinds of wrestling holds there are, the *paidotribai* will show, laying down the principles of the opportune moment (*kairous*), the attack, the ex-tent of practice, and the rules for defending oneself or for breaking through another's defense" (14.269). About seven centuries had passed since Gorgias "failed" to define *kairos*—*Peri Gymnastikēs* is dated around 220 CE—yet the impossibility of detailing *kairos* remains, as attention to *kairos* is incorporated into Philostratus' training regimen. In other words, knowledge of the right time, opening, and the right way is inexo-rably bound with knowledge of opponents, methods of attack, types of holds.

The ease with which athletic training illustrates and incorporates *kai-ros* helps account for why Gorgias' student Isocrates turned to gym-nastics in order to demonstrate how a "program" for sophistic rhetoric takes shape. As Isocrates figures it, *paidotribai* instruct their students "in the postures which have been devised for bodily contests," while the teachers of *philosophia* impart "forms of discourse." Just as Philostratus would do centuries later, Isocrates links the teaching of moves to the teaching of situations, for along with instruction in basic moves, teach-ers of both gymnastics and rhetoric

> again exercise the students and habituate them to hard work, and then compel them to combine (*suneirein*) everything they have learned, in order that they may grasp them more firmly (*bebaioteron kataschōsi*) and bring their notions (*doxais*) in closer touch with the occasions (*tōn kairōn*) for applying them—I say "notions" for no sys-tem of knowledge is able to cover these occasions, since in all cir-cumstances they escape our knowledge (*epistēmas*). (*Antidosis* 184)

In Isocrates' view, *kairos* thus flees epistemology, eluding the systematic definition desired by Dionysius of Halicarnassus.

If *kairos* cannot be known, then how might *kairos* be taught? One way, as Isocrates suggests, is to foster a kind of synthetic, embodied training that relies on the repeated production of encounters—this sort of training will be the focus of the next chapter. Another way to teach kairos, however, is to offer an illustrative kairotic body—perhaps such a body would come in the form of a *pharmakon*, a beguiling incantation, or a performative speech such as Gorgias' *Helen*. Or perhaps it would be cast in bronze, a sculpted rendition of the god Kairos himself. In other words, the sculptor Lysippos seemed to know early on what Dionysius of Halicarnassus would never realize: a kairotic body may be the most apt form such a "lesson" can take.

❄ 4 ❄

Phusiopoiesis

The Arts of Training

With *mētis* and *kairos* as central concepts for ancient rhetorical practices, then training, as suggested toward the end of the last chapter, might take the form of exemplary display (thus emphasizing the teaching body), or, as suggested in chapter 2, would focus on the body's capacity to "think" (emphasizing the learning body). To be sure, at the heart of both *mētis* and *kairos* is the notion of bodily transformation—the capacity to respond and transform in different situations. As this chapter will suggest, the cultivation of a capacity to transform is an important component of sophistic training practice, and the body figures directly into the dynamics of training.

At the beginning of Plato's *Protagoras,* the title character reminds Socrates that the art of sophistry has a long and various history, and is often characterized by disguise (*proschēma poieisthai kai prokaluptesthai*):

> Sometimes of poetry, as in the case of Homer, Hesiod, and Simonides; sometimes of initiation rites and prophecies, as did Orpheus, Musaeus and their sects; and sometimes too, I have observed, of athletics, as with Iccus of Tarentum and another still living—as great a sophist as any—Herodicus of Selymbria, originally of Megara; and music was the disguise employed by Agathocles, a great sophist, Pythocleides of Ceos, and many more. (*Protagoras* 316d–e)

While Protagoras uses these examples to distinguish himself as someone who did not rely on a disguise, or "outer covering," for his art of sophistry, all of the instantiations of sophistic *technē* cited here—poetry, music, athletics, and sports medicine (Herodicus of Selymbria was an early practitioner of medicine for athletes)—nonetheless deal with a kind of education, a shaping of the body-mind complex. As the character Protagoras puts it a few lines earlier, all these arts hold the promise of self-improvement (*beltious esomenous,* "becoming better") attained through students' "linking to" (*suneinai*) those sophists who practice them.

The age of Protagoras (known more commonly as the age of Pericles) was a time when the "spirit of *technē*"[1] was spreading through Athens. The sophistic arts mentioned by Protagoras, as the previous two chapters suggest, were imbued with a cunning sensibility (*mētis*) as well as a kind of kairotic deployment. While training in these arts took many different forms relevant to the production of musical, poetic, athletic, or rhetorical aptitudes the general direction was a kind of self-stylization, of making oneself better and more capable in some regard.

At first glance, these arts seem to fall under the category developed so lucidly by Michel Foucault in regard to the ancients; they are "arts of existence," *technē tou biou* (1988: 44–45). Foucault uses this phrase to indicate

> those intentional and voluntary actions by which men not only set themselves rules of conduct, but also seek to transform themselves, to change themselves in their singular being, and to make their life into an *oeuvre* that carries certain aesthetic values and meets certain stylistic criteria. (1990: 10–11)

Foucault's description is written almost entirely in the reflexive middle voice, whereby men "seek to transform themselves." In other words, a major requirement for transformation is the "seeking out" motivated by a desire to cultivate strategies that will produce oneself differently. Such a seeking is, however, accompanied by a concomitant submitting: active submission is thus a necessary first step for transformation. But even more than that, values and styles cultivated by such actions work to create capacities, flexible bodies of work. Insofar as these training practices produce a capacity for transformation, arts of existence, especially in the sophistic milieu under consideration here, might be more aptly construed as "arts of becoming."

For Protagoras, active submission manifests itself in a choice to "join with" (*suneinai*) a particular teacher, as the itinerant sophist encourages youths to "drop their other connections, either with their families or with foreigners, both old and young, and to join one's own circle, with the promise of improving them by this connection with oneself" (316c–d). Indeed, the impetus for the entire dialogue is young Hippocrates' "intention (*melleis*) to submit (*paraschein*)" himself to a sophist (312c). In other words, a certain dynamic necessarily precedes the kind of transformation promised by sophistic *technai*.

Moving among general theories of training, this chapter will delineate several dynamics and directions produced by these programs for transformation, these ancient arts of becoming.

Arts of Flesh

The fifth-century Hippocratic treatise *Regimen,* or *Peri Diatēs,* offers observations on bodily regimen and training and usefully elaborates an ancient *technē* of daily existence. The Hippocratics functioned, after all, as the contemporary authorities on bodies and their care, and so medical perspectives on daily existence form a crucial backdrop for any sort of bodily training. The *diata* of the treatise's title generally means "a way of living" or "a mode of life," and the text encourages those specializing in the medical art to pay attention to general modes of existence rather than to focus on conditions of ill health.

According to the author, it is necessary for a physician who will offer counsel on daily regimen to know the constitution of the human body, the forces within it (1.2.1–10), as well as "the power (*dunamin*) possessed by all the food and drinks of our regimen, both according to nature and by means of force of human art (*technēn anthrōpinēn*)" (1.2.10–15). In other words, the physician's task is to attend to capacities and tendencies—the capacities of particular bodies to be affected in particular ways by forces of nature and art. Such an approach is highly contingent on the situation at hand and relies on a kind of kairotic know-how: "For it is necessary to know both how one ought to lessen the power of these when they are strong by nature, and when they are weak to apply strength via art, seizing each opportunity (*ho kairos*) as it occurs" (1.2.10). The text's physician is thus one who attends to and tinkers with a variety of forces—corporeal, material, technical—in an attempt to produce and maintain a healthy, regulated body.

But regulation here does not mean fixity. Rather, the strategies and practices (read: "arts") outlined in *Regimen* are based on the assumption that change will happen, as the text is targeted toward "those who of necessity live a haphazard life (*eikē ton bion*)" (3.69.1). The word *eikē*, here translated "haphazard," entails a kind of randomness or movement without a plan and implies that a "regimen" or general mode of existence has many variables—food, drink, exercise, general condition of health—that meet with changing practices from day to day. Thus, in this text, the very concept of regulation is an emergent one; an ideal art would enable a medical practitioner to respond to changing circumstances productively.

Foucault's consideration of the Hippocratic texts underscores their emphasis on *use* for a particular person. As Foucault sees it, "The usefulness of a regimen lay precisely in the possibility it gave individuals to face different situations" (1990: 105). The treatise, then, provides a diagram of transformative forces—diseases, bodies, substances, exercises—and their potentialities. In other words, the author of *Regimen*, intensely interested in relations, responses, and effects, seeks to elaborate a technique of regimen development to accompany and facilitate the optimal condition of these forces.

Corporeal Production: Fire and Water

Regimen contains long descriptions of various foods, drinks, and herbs and their effects on the body's constitution—whether they cool or warm, moisten or dry the body, and whether they "pass" well or not. These catalogues are followed by a consideration of practices; descriptions of the effects of sleeping (2.60), vomiting (2.59), oiling (2.57), exercising (2.61), and bathing, the last of which reads as follows:

> As for baths, their properties are as follows. Fresh water moistens and refreshes, for it gives moisture to the body. A salt bath warms and dries, for the condition of heat draws the moisture from the body. Hot baths, when taken fasting, wither and cool, for through their warmth they carry the moisture from the body, while as the flesh is emptied of its moisture the body is cooled. Taken after a meal, they warm and moisten, as they expand to a greater bulk the moisture already existing in the body. Cold baths have an opposite effect. To an empty body they give a certain amount of heat; after a meal they take away moisture and fill with their dryness, which is cold. Being unwashed dries, using up moisture, and likewise being unoiled. (2.57; trans. adapted from Jones 1953)

This passage on bathing, in the typical style of *Regimen*, details the bath's effects in relation to many variables—type and temperature of water, condition of the body, and so forth. In other words, the practice of bathing, like the other practices treated in *Regimen*, cannot be considered separately from its circumstance. Such an approach sets up a fluid set of practical principles, a compendium of tendencies. Moreover, in this passage, as in the rest of the treatise, the author focuses on the calibration of the body's temperature and moisture level, or what he calls "fire" and "water," two of the ancient bodily elements.[2]

As the author describes early in *Regimen*, all animals (humans included) are thought to be comprised of fire and water. The two elements work in relation to each other, and neither can overpower the body:

> The fire, as it advances to the limit of the water, leaves behind nourishment, and then it is turned back where it is likely to grow; the water, as it advances to the limit of the fire, leaves behind motion, and then stops here. When it stops it is no longer in possession of force, and immediately it meets with the fire, which devours its nourishment. (1.3.14–19)

Regimen's author thus articulates a belief prevalent in the Hippocratic tradition as well as in other philosophies based on humoral theories: the takeover of one humor or element would mean disease or death (Jones 1953: xlviii).

Fire and water thus exist and move in responsive relation: fire gleans nourishment from water; water, kinetic heat from fire. Both enable the other's movement, and here the movement is what enables life:

> For as never staying in the same condition, but always changing to this or to that, separating off from these elements things that are necessarily dissimilar. So of all things nothing is destroyed, and nothing emerges that did not exist before. Things change merely by mingling (*summisgomena*) and being separated (*diakrinomena*). (1.4.10–14)

Here, mingling (*summisgomena*) comes from the middle verb *summignumi*, which may be translated "mix together, commingle"; "join forces" or "form an alliance, as in armies"; "have sexual intercourse with"; "meet, as in communicate"; and "meet in a close fight," in a hostile sense.

All these nuances of *summignumi* become useful when considering the bodily relation between fire and water and the production of change described in *Regimen*. New material is not introduced; rather, the movement from distinguishability (*diakrinomena*—from *diakrinō*, "to separate, to decompose into elemental parts, to remove or distinguish") to an indistinguishable alliance constitutes the very production of change. Fire and water, insofar as they comprise humans' bodies and souls,[3] were considered in the Hippocratic tradition to be the very material of transformation: "all things, both human and divine, are in flux, exchanging upwards and downwards" (1.5.1–3). These exchanges, or "minglings," as the author prefers to call them, take the form of struggle:

> Into man go parts of parts and wholes of wholes, containing a mixture of fire and water, some to take and others to give. Those that take make more, those that give make less. Men saw wood; while one pulls, the other pushes. But they do the same thing, and while making less, they make more. Such is the nature (*phusis*) of man. (1.6.1–6)

Even human bodies, then, are constituted by an agonistic mingling, by an alliance of forces—with fire and water being the most basic. This axiom emerges most explicitly in an extended description of the struggle between these two elements. According to the Hippocratic text, fire generally cuts paths to nourishment, or water (1.9.28). From there it blazes new passages to the places most abundant with water:

> Hence the fire issued forth, since it had no nourishment, and made passages for the breath and the supplying and distribution of nourishment. The fire shut up in the rest of the body made itself three passages, the moistest part of the fire being in those places called the hollow veins. And in the middle of these the remaining water becomes compacted and congealed. It is called flesh. (1.9.34–38)

The Hippocratic tradition thus held that flesh—the body itself—emerges from an active, combinatory exchange: from alliances and separations. Corporeality is thus an effect of a type of *agōn* of the variety described in chapter 1: the productive encounter between forces. It is the physician's job to "tinker" with these agonistic forces or provoke them in particular directions to try to produce the most balanced, flexible disposition.

Shaping Bodies

It becomes apparent throughout *Regimen* that the agonistic constitution of human bodies provides the basis for kairotic theories of regimen development and training. In fact, immediately following the discussion of fire and water and emergent flesh, the author of *Regimen* explicitly invokes the *paidotribēs,* or gymnastic trainer, as a wielder of fire and water:

> Craftsmen melt the iron with fire, constraining the fire by blowing; the nourishment it has already is taken away; when they have made it rare, they beat it and weld it; and with the nourishment of other water it grows strong. In this way is a man treated by his trainer (*paidotribou*). By fire the nourishment he has already is taken away, under the constraining blowing. As he is made rare, he is struck, rubbed, and purged. On the application of water from elsewhere he becomes strong. (1.13.1–10)

The analogy here is quite explicit: the trainee aligns with the iron that gets shaped by craftsman or trainer (*paidotribēs*). But the way the analogy unfolds reveals a good deal about the method and use of training. According to this passage, the first step in shaping iron or athletes is to rarify the material, to make it thin or porous, less dense (*araioō*). In other words, by attending to the bodily—fire and water—the craftsman or *paidotribēs* can render material malleable. After rarification of the iron, the craftsmen "beat" (*paiousi*) and "weld" (*sunelaunousin*) it. The verb *paiousi* (*paiō*), here translated "beat," usually means "smite," or to drive or dash one thing against the other. The verb *sunelaunousin* (*sunelaunō*), on the other hand, suggests fusion, as it means "to drive or hammer together." *Sunelaunō* may also be translated "to match in combat or set to fight." The translation of this verb as "weld," while it captures nicely the connecting force of the Greek, loses a bit of the brute force necessary to produce such a connection.

When the analogy is carried over to the *paidotribēs,* however, the writer makes use of a different set of verbs: the athlete is "struck" (*koptetai*), "rubbed" (*tribetai*), and "purged" (*kathairetai*). The first verb parallels the "beating" of iron, but has a slightly different force. While *paiousi* suggests a forceful striking, *koptō* suggests a beating or a stamping, as in the making of metal into coins. In other words, when "stamped" in this way, one is shaped for a particular purpose or use. The verb for "rubbed," *tribetai,* is the same as that found in *paidotribēs,* one who educates or trains children. The distance from "rubbing" or "wearing down" of an object to "training" or "educating" isn't too far at all. This verb also appears in Plato's *Sophist* (as discussed in chapter 2), where the wily fox found his way in the dark through "practice" (*tribēs*). Here, *tribō,* with its forces of "wearing," "practice," and "exercise" suggests a necessary repetition of actions. To follow the Hippocratic author's analogy, in order to produce a particular shape, one cannot simply "strike" the iron, but one must strike it in a particular way—more than once—to produce the desired shape. The final verb in the set, *kathairetai,* is translated "purged," and suggests a kind of cleansing or clearing out of the older elements or "nourishment," a kind of "purification" through purging.

The ancient art of physical training is therefore formulated as a force which, when placed in relation to the bodily forces of fire and water, actually reconfigures the body's composition, producing corporeal transformation. Such transformation, as noted earlier, must be accompanied by a desire for change; in this way, provocation and seduction together help produce the dynamics necessary for effective training.

Phusiopoiesis

At work in these *Regimen* passages is the notion of what I'm calling *phusiopoiesis,* creation of a person's nature. I take this term from Democritean fragment 33: "Nature and instruction (*didachē*) are similar; for instruction shapes (*metarusmoi*) the man, and in shaping, produces his nature (*phusiopoiei*)." Here, Democritus provides a defining term for what is described so lucidly in *Regimen*'s analogy between the *paidotribēs* and the iron maker: the body's constitution can be remolded so that it is more suitable for further training. The term used by Democritus (*phusiopoiei*) thus fuses two critical concepts: *phusis,* or nature, and *poieō,* commonly known to mean "make or do," "produce," or "create," and often used in the context of particular *technai* such as carpentry, medicine, and writing or speaking.

Phusiopoiesis holds important implications for the quality and direction of Presocratic educational practices. Indeed, *phusiopoietic* practices depend on dynamics of submission and seduction that manifest themselves in a number of ways. What follows will detail some of these directions by considering the forces at work in ancient bodily training practices.

A Second Nature

It is well known that ancient philosophers and scientists wrote more about the notion of nature (*phusis*) than about almost any other concept. A number of Presocratics wrote treatises entitled *Peri Phuseō*, or "On Nature"; among them were Xenophon, Heraclitus, Gorgias, and Epicurus.

As is commonly observed, translation of *phusis* as "nature" excludes some of the various dimensions of the ancient word, even as it imports contemporary assumptions about the category, as in the word that opposes and helps define "culture," or that which is produced.[4] It is therefore important to emphasize that while the ancient concept of *phusis* carried meanings that would fall on the "nature" side of the contemporary nature/culture divide, the word also suggests "temperament" and "character," and contains a common connotation of "growth."

Phusis thus already implies a kind of capacity for change, the force encapsulated by *phusiopoiesis*. As William Arthur Heidel points out, Aristotle's approach to *phusis* draws out the implications of Presocratic treatises on nature (1910: 108). In a discussion of *phusis* in *Metaphysics,* Aristotle quotes Empedocles as saying that "not one existing thing is nature, but only mixture and separation of that which has been mixed; *phusis* is the name given these by men" (*Metaphysics* 1015a). This observation parallels that made in *Regimen* about somatic humors, whereby "things change merely by mingling and being separated"—the saying is attributed to Anaxagoras also (Jones 1953: 245 n. 1) and appears to have been something of a commonplace among the Presocratics.

After further consideration of the category of *phusis* in relation to these Presocratic tenets, Aristotle concludes:

> From what has been said, then, the primary and authoritative sense of "nature" is those things that have in themselves as such a cause of motion; for the material is called "nature" because it is capable of receiving the nature, and the processes of becoming and growing are called "nature" because they are motions produced by it. And the beginning of motion is somehow inherent in natural objects, either potentially (*dunamei*) or actually. (*Metaphysics* 1015a15–20)

In other words, *phusis* is both the capacity for and the effect of movement and change, most especially in the "disposition and temperament" dimensions of the word.

The disposition and temperament aspects of *phusis* suggest a link to the ancient concepts of *ethos* (habit), *ēthos* (disposition, character), and *hexis* (state, condition, habit of the body). In the *Rhetoric*, Aristotle explains the close relation between habit (*ethos*) and nature (*phusis*):

> Movement into a natural state is thus necessarily pleasurable for the most part, and especially whenever a natural process has recovered its own natural state. And habits [are pleasurable]; for the habitual has already become, as it were, natural; for habit is something like nature (*gar ti to ethos tē phusei*). (*Rhetoric* 1.11.1370a4; trans. Kennedy)

Here, Aristotle suggests that habits become so ingrained in a person that they become almost instinctual responses and most closely approximate a "natural" state.

Along the same lines, in the *Nicomachean Ethics*, Aristotle usefully elaborates the relation between *phusis* and *ethos* by placing them in succession. After delineating two kinds of *aretē*—intellectual and moral—Aristotle goes on to describe how nature first installs certain tendencies and habit subsequently develops those tendencies, thus explaining the way *phusis* and *ethos* work in tandem:

> The *aretas*, therefore, emerge in us neither beside nature nor before nature, but rather nature produces in us the capacity to exhibit them, perfecting them by means of habit (*teleioumenois de dia tou ethous*). (*Nicomachean Ethics* 2.1.1103a)

In this passage, Aristotle explicitly renders *phusis* and habit in a complementary, successive relation. Habit draws out the virtuous actions that nature makes one tend toward, bringing them to completion (*teleioumenois*), perfecting them through repetitive practice. Through habit, therefore, a "second nature" emerges.

Given its relation to habit and *aretē*, it is not surprising that Isocrates places "nature" foremost on the list of necessary ingredients for rhetorical training (c.f. Too 2000: 46–47; Shorey 1909). But he elaborates the category precisely as *potentiality* and links it so immediately with practice that the two are mutually constitutive. Isocrates' ideal pupil thus comes equipped with a mind (*psuchēn*) that is able (*dunamenēn*) to find and to learn and to work hard and to remember what it learns, and also a voice and a clarity of mouth that are able to persuade the audience, not only by words alone, but by harmonious words, yet he would undertake these qualities without producing a mark of shamelessness, but preparing the mind in the midst of moderation in this way so that it has as much confidence making speeches to all citizens as in reflecting to himself. (*Antidosis* 189–90)

Isocrates' discussion of natural ability merges with his discussion of practice or training, and he concludes that "if either one of these factors [i.e., *phusis* or practice] would make one powerful in speaking and managing affairs, both of them arising in the same person might render a man insurpassable by others" (*Antidosis* 191). In other words, for Isocrates, the students must be capable of being transformed—of being fashioned in the same way that the *Regimen* author portrays with the athlete-as-iron analogy.

What's more, Isocrates' reflections on the combination of nature and practice extend an observation attributed to Protagoras: "Teaching requires nature and practice (*phuseōs kai askēseōs*)" (DK 80 B3). That *phusis* is malleable and therefore trainable is one of the main tenets of sophistic thought, and is best illustrated in Plato's *Protagoras* when the character Protagoras argues that *aretē* can be taught.

As Werner Jaeger points out in his three-volume study of ancient *paideia*, the sophists' conclusion about the flexibility of *phusis* "is an attempt at a synthesis of the old opposition between aristocratic paideia and rationalism: it abandons the aristocratic idea that character and morality can be inherited by blood, but not acquired" (Jaeger 1967: 306). As this study suggests, however, rationalism is not necessarily the sophists' additive component. Rather, the sophists and Isocrates gather their notion of a malleable *phusis* from Archaic models of education, leaning heavily on poetic, musical, and athletic training as models for and necessary partners to rhetorical training, models that depend on a bodily acquisition of disposition and styles of thought. As such, the Archaic educational practices upon which the sophists draw are not merely guided by rational modes of learning but depend upon the cultivation of bodily desire, a general kind of readiness to learn, provocation, and, at times, pain and erotics. What follows will treat each of these in turn.

In the dialogue *Protagoras,* the old sophist elaborates a whole network of Archaic educational practices, pointing out the subtle ways in which training in verse, music, and athletics prepares the mind-body complex for its role in the *polis.* According to the character Protagoras, the teacher, or *grammatēs,* provides young boys "with works of good poets to read as they sit in class"; the students thus examine the verses closely and learn them by heart (*ekmanthanein*). It is in the poems that the youths "meet with many admonitions, many descriptions and praises and eulogies of good men in times past, that the boy in envy may imitate (*mimētai*) them and yearn to become them (*oregētai toioutos genesthai*)" (*Protagoras* 326a).[5]

Later we will return to the function of imitation in education, but for now, the crucial phrasing here is *oregētai toioutos genesthai,* the production of desire to become something else. *Oregētai,* here translated as "yearn," also holds the sense of "to stretch oneself out to," or to reach for. The character Protagoras thus suggests that subjection to the works of "good poets" (namely Homer, Hesiod, and the like) functions to spark an interest in self-transformation and thus marks the capacity for *phusiopoiesis.*

Training in music works in a similar fashion, as youths "are taught the works of another set of good poets, the songmakers, while the master accompanies them on the harp." Moreover, Protagoras continues, the music teachers "insist on (*anagkazousin*) the boys' souls familiarizing themselves (*oikeiousthai*) with the rhythms and scales, that they may gain in gentleness, and by advancing in rhythmic and harmonic grace may be efficient in speech and action; for the whole of man's life requires the graces of rhythm and harmony" (*Protagoras* 326b). Here, the middle participle *oikeiousthai,* rooted in the familiar term for house or dwelling (*oikos*), suggests that the rhythms and scales come to inhabit the young *psychai;* quite literally "moving in."[6]

Musical education cultivated a rhythmic way of moving through the world, a style of engagement that fanned out into the "whole of life" (*pas bios*). And, most important, according to the character Protagoras, is that "over and above all this, people send their sons to a trainer (*paidotribou*), that having improved their bodies they may serve their minds, which are now in fit condition, and that they may not be forced by bodily faults to play the coward in wars and other duties" (*Protago-*

ras 326b–c). Just as training in music provides youths with a sense of rhythmic movement and gentleness, athletic training promises to instill the values of strength and bravery.

For this study's purposes, though, the most important feature of Protagoras' description lies in the language of desire production; the way in which reading the work of the great poets caused the young boys to yearn for—to reach themselves out to—a set of training practices. In this way, early education cultivated a readiness for more training.

A READINESS

Timing is a critical indicator of the possibility of *phusiopoiesis*. Another Democritean fragment suggests that there are certain times in life when one's *phusis* is more malleable: "There is a sagacity (*xunesis*) of the young, and a nonsagacity of the aged. It is not time (*chronos*) that teaches practical wisdom (*phronein*), but timely training and nature (*hōraiē trophē kai phusis*)" (DK 68 B183). The word for perceptiveness here, *xunesis* (also *sunesis*), has the general meaning of "union," but it can also mean a type of intelligence that has to do with quickness of comprehension. *Xunesis* thus suggests a certain attunement, much along the lines of a kairotic disposition (as discussed in the last chapter).

It is this faculty of keen perceptiveness, thought by Democritus to be present in youths, that must be "tapped" at the right time. This fragment thus upends the abiding ancient notion that wisdom is tied to duration of life experiences, as suggested, for example, in the figure of old, wise Nestor. It is also important to note here that the wisdom is *phronēsis*, a kind of contingent practical wisdom in one's affairs, a partner-term to *mētis*. Such awareness is distinct from "knowledge" in that it cannot be *accumulated* over time (*chronos*), but rather must be developed early on, when one has a certain perceptive quality, a kind of readiness.

This notion of the importance of readiness in training inhabits sophistic thought. Isocrates, in the ethical treatise *To Demonicus,* echoes the Democritean perspective on a certain quality of mind:

> I see that luck is on our side and that the present opportunity shares with us in our struggle (*kairon sunagōnizomenon*); for you have set your heart on education (*paideuein*) and I profess to educate; you are ripe for philosophy (*akmē philosophein*), and I instruct students of philosophy. (*To Demonicus* 1.3)

The time is right. Demonicus is ready, *akmē*. He is eager for training, and the treatise, sent to Demonicus as a gift (*ton logon dōron*) and a token of friendship (*philia*), joins him with Isocrates in his quest for education. The openness of his heart (*epithumeis*) combined with the acceptance of the gift confirms his willingness to be taught, to become a friend of Isocrates: *phusiopoiesis* has begun.

This quality of readiness binds training with *kairos* as opportunity or opening. Just as the regimen designer must attend to the immediate circumstances of daily practices, the trainer/teacher remains attuned to the subject's capacity for learning, or the desire to transform. At the same time, a prospective student must open the self in order to enter into a relation with the teacher.

As discussed in chapter 3, however, in the context of education, *kairos* eludes programmatic qualities. That is, phusiopoietic *kairos* cannot be articulated as "steps" for improvement, but rather emerges among a variety of dynamic forces. This emergence happens in a way that troubles a notion of an individual making conscious choices—in other words, it is not simply the student's agency, whereby he "seeks out" training, nor is it only the teacher/trainer's agency, whereby he seduces the student to yearn for transformation.[7] The dynamic is more responsive, more mutual, and at times less conscious than such a description would suggest.

In other words, *phusiopoiesis* is a dynamic of stylization that emerges *between* teacher and student. Here, the kairotic opening happens on the level of the self. An opening up of the self/other distinction facilitates a kind of reciprocal bond between teacher and student guided by complimentary capacities: "you have set your heart on education and I profess to educate; you are ripe for philosophy, and I instruct students of philosophy." An exchange occurs, a mutual questing ignites. Yet simply noting the convergence of desires as necessary for *phusiopoeisis* does not do much to diagnose the dynamics at work. What follows, then, will examine three distinct yet related phusiopoietic relations crucial for ancient training practices (friendship, pain, and erotics), and will consider how these relations helped style bodily arts of becoming.

PROVOCATION

The pedagogic dimension of friendship invoked by Isocrates should not be taken lightly. The relationship between teacher and student depends on a kind of friendship, a mutual commitment to each other in a quest for improvement. Ancient friendship, which may be characterized following David Konstan as "a mutually intimate, loyal, and loving bond" (1997: 1), thus introduces vital, affective ties between two or more people.

Konstan, drawing on anthropological language, labels friendship "achieved" rather than "ascribed" (1997: 1, 55), and argues convincingly that ancient friendship was predicated on "affection and generosity rather than on obligatory reciprocity" (5). The achievement of intimacy called *philia*, further, produces something altogether new. In this regard, phusiopoietic *philia* approximates what has been called *allopoiesis*,[8] the production of something other than itself, in that something else—desire, knowledge, gifts, cultural change, revelations of peculiarity—is produced through a bond with someone else. Such a poetic economy entails precisely what Isocrates refers to in his treatise to Demonicus and what Protagoras refers to in the context of early education—an opening of the self out onto the other.[9]

The *Regimen*'s description of the *paidotribēs*'s relation to the athlete-in-training most explicitly depicts this kind of concomitant entrusting and shaping from the outside. But it is important to note that the outside here—in this case the *paidotribēs*—is part of the athlete's training ecology. That is, as soon as the athlete opens up to the other (the *paidotribēs*), the distinction between inside and outside becomes less perceptible. The fire-water of the body yields to the fire-wielding *paidotribēs*; the submission effects a bond of *philia* that produces the self anew. The *paidotribēs*, in turn, provokes the trainee by encouraging practices and movements in ways that will produce the bodily *aretē* discussed in chapter 1. Thus, both athletic and sophistic pedagogy depend on a contractual *philia*, a tacit agreement to transform.[10]

NO PAIN, NO CHANGE

Recalling the violent language of *Regimen*, wherein the *paidotribēs* "beats, rubs, and purges" the athlete, how can *phusiopoiesis* be an instantiation of *philia*? That is to say, doesn't friendship entail a mutual direction, or at the very least, equal ground? The ancient educative relationship was more than just "tough love"; it functioned instead as a ritual relation with elements of pain and suffering.

The active submission of the student, the cultivation of "readiness" discussed earlier, might be read as a consent to—even a demand for—

painful subjection. When the teacher is seduced to oblige the student's openness, an alliance is formed. More important, however, is that the training itself becomes a responsive, reciprocal relation: the athlete and the athlete's body suggest directions for training, and the trainer pushes in these directions while provoking others.

In the context of athletic training, the role of the *paidotribēs* requires the trainer to take on a two-fold role, one demonstrative, one corrective, with the latter often taking a punitive form. These two roles are depicted quite commonly in ancient artistic renderings of the *paidotribēs*. The *paidotribēs* appears in training scenes (see figure 4.1, third figure from left) wearing a long cloak and carrying a long, forked stick, a *lugos*, a pliant, forked stick made of willow or fennel stalks (Crowther 1988: 73). The trainer would remove his cloak only in order to demonstrate movements to the athletes-in-training, and the *lugos* served as a tool of correction: if an athlete's body was slightly out of position, the *paidotribēs* would use the stick to intervene during practice, guiding the body in a particular way.

Such intervention was likely not a matter of "nudging"—indeed, the stick was probably used more as a tool for punishment for inattentiveness or incorrect movements (Marrou 1956: 392; Gardiner 1910: 304), as suggested by the actions of the *paidotribēs* in figures 4.2 and 4.3. Figure 4.2, a scene from a red-figure vase, depicts a pankration lesson, wherein the *paidotribēs* uses the forked rod to intervene in the pankratiasts' practice. At the left, a boy prepares a boxing thong.

Figures 4.3 and 4.4 also show the *paidotribēs* putting his forked stick to use. Figure 4.3 shows a pankration training scene with the *paidotribēs* off to the right, stick raised to a striking position. The pankratiast on the right is gouging his opponent's eye, and the *paidotribēs* is about to flog the offender.[11] Figure 4.4, on the other hand, shows the *paidotribēs* using his stick to correct jumping form, as the jumper, holding *halterēs* (jumping weights), is in midair.

Pain and suffering were not, however, restricted to athletic training.[12] In a discussion of disciplinary pedagogy, Too notes how Isocrates' imitative pedagogy offers the teacher as "the mold (*tupos*) from which the claylike students will emerge" (2000: 44). The word *tupos*, as Too demonstrates, is not limited to "exemplar," as its verb form, *tuptō*, goes further to encapsulate the action necessary to "strike," "beat," or "pound" out the desired result, as in the contexts of pottery, coin making, or fighting. The resulting "impression" is lasting and material.

As Too and Marrou both observe, the role of physical punitive action in education was tacitly invoked by the use, in Hellenistic grammar handbooks, of the verb *tuptō* as a paradigmatic verb of regular declension. As Too puts it, "the verb provides a constant reminder that the student who is slack will be disciplined by beating" (2000: 45; see also Marrou 1956: 221–22, 238). As any student of language knows (especially students of ancient Greek!), the repetitive practice necessary for learning grammatical forms on its own is enough to constitute a kind of stamping or beating.

In addition to the obvious repetitive practice, which will be treated later, pain functions as a critical element in the educative relation; Aristotle puts it quite succinctly: "learning [happens] by aid of pain" (*meta lupēs*) (*Politics* 8.1339a28). Pain therefore works as a facilitator of transformation, an enabler of sorts. This is not to say, however, that pain *is* pleasure, but rather, that pain functions as a requisite to gratification—pain is an enabler. In other words, pain acts to produce one in a particular way (emphasis on "produce" as verb, not product).

Pain in the teacher-student relationship therefore approximates the athletic questing discussed in chapter 1, where the victory received less emphasis and the questing—a seeking of the identity of "victorious athlete" which depends on a constant deferral of the identity—became the focus.

What pain enables in the training matrix, then, is a continual "opening up" of the athletic subject, the production of a bond between *paidotribēs* and athlete, and hence between the athletic body and the moves and postures it acquires. It is through constant and repeated subjection to the teacher, whether in the context of intense and insistent grammar lessons, oratorical exhibitions, or the *paidotribēs'* cloakless demonstrations and relentless forked stick. In all these instances, pain is transformative, and was therefore deemed, as Aristotle suggests, a necessary accompaniment to education.

EROTICS

It is well known that the relation between ancient teacher and student often moved into the realm of *eros*. Such movement was not merely "incidental," nor was it uncommon.

As two key studies—Claude Calame's *Poetics of Eros in Ancient Greece* (1999) and Michel Foucault's *Use of Pleasure* (1990)—demonstrate, the ancients devoted a good deal of time to defining the domain of erotics

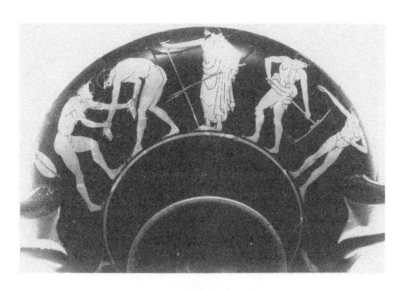

FIGURE 4.1
Palaestra scene, from an Athenian red-figure kylix (cup): Ashmolean
Museum 1914.729, side A. © Ashmolean Museum, Oxford.

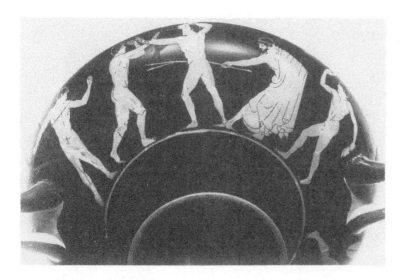

FIGURE 4.2
Scene showing a pankration lesson, from an Athenian red-figure kylix:
Ashmolean Museum 1914.729, side B. © Ashmolean Museum, Oxford.

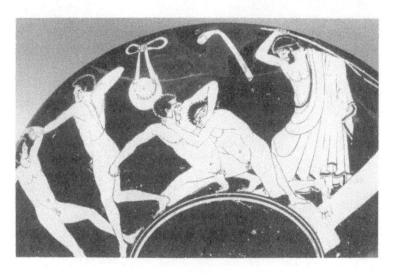

FIGURE 4.3
Scene showing pankratiasts, from an Athenian red-figure kylix:
British Museum E 78. © British Museum, London.

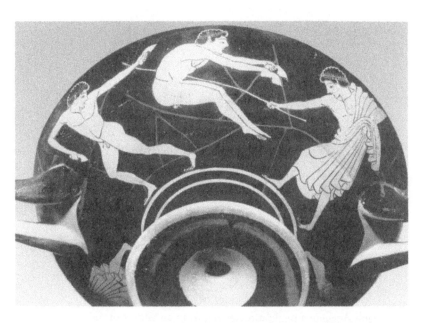

FIGURE 4.4
Scene showing jumping training, from an Athenian red-figure kylix:
Museum of Fine Arts 01.8020. © Museum of Fine Arts, Boston.

between men and boys. Foucault also points out that such relations weren't confined to educational practice, though they certainly occurred in educative contexts.[13] Still, as Foucault's study suggests, erotics between men and boys, with all its conventions, rules of conduct, and "games of delays and obstacles designed to put off the moment of closure" (1988: 197), had its own domain of *paideia* (see Bremmer 1990). In other words, the domain of male erotics had a distinctive stylistics, and these were demonstrated and perpetuated in the relations themselves.

Even as erotics had its own dimension of pedagogy, pedagogy had dimensions of erotics. In some ways, the pleasures of erotics can be seen, like pain in the teacher-student relation, as another enabler of training—indeed, the active submission necessary for *phusiopoiesis* can be seen as a response to seduction. Such seduction may or may not have erotic overtones, but in ancient Athens it often did. The Greek gymnasium, with its open spaces and nude exercisers, along with its function as both a training site and a place of leisure, was itself a space for seduction. The statue of Eros placed at the entrance to the gymnasium of Athens offers what Calame calls "the most striking evidence of the place reserved for Eros in spaces designed for exercise and physical education" (1999: 101). Chapter 5 will examine the gymnasium more closely, but for now, suffice it to say that the gymnasium and the palaestra (the wrestling school) are often invoked in Greek literature and art as the loci for male-male erotics.[14]

But the gymnasium wasn't just a "free-for-all." As Foucault explains, erotics between men and boys had its own precisely demarcated domain of ethics as well; in order to remain within acceptable conventions, Greek men had to take care only to enter into sexual relations with their subordinates, which included women, slaves, and those younger or "lesser born" than they. Ancient sexual practices thus depended on a kind of asymmetry and operated on what John J. Winkler refers to as "a calculus of profit" (1990: 37), wherein one gives (submits) and the other takes. As a result, as K. J. Dover points out, evidence of same-age men engaging in sexual activity is virtually nonexistent (1978: 16).

The result, in Calame's concise formulation, was "a relationship doomed to asymmetry" (1999: 29). This asymmetry manifested itself in language as well; men and boys who engaged in erotic activity were not referred to individually as "lovers," but rather each had a name which designated—often quite literally—his position in the relationship. The term used for the boy is *eromenos,* the passive participle of *eran,* "be in love with" or "have a passionate desire for," and may therefore be rendered "the beloved." The man or senior partner, on the other hand, was referred to more generally as the *erastēs,* the lover, a term which blends with "admirer" as well.[15]

Still, male-to-male erotics was also governed by an ascetic principle of self-control; as Winkler notes, it was considered good for a man to be "stronger than himself (*kreittōn heautou*), able to manage and control his various appetites" (1990: 50). This principle did not, however, dictate total abstention, but rather an attention to specificity, a certain "stylization" of erotic practices, as Foucault puts it, and a concomitant valorization of the relation (1990: 245).

Here we can see an *agōn* emerging; one struggles with oneself in the context of *erōs,* as one attends to the appropriateness of erotic relations with a certain person in particular settings. Like so many other practices elaborated in this study, then, the ethics of erotics depended on circumstances, *kairos,* or what Foucault calls a "politics of timeliness."

As Dover points out, Xenophon's version of an appropriate male-male erotic relationship depended on its connections to education (1978: 202). To be sure, in the passage Dover cites from Xenophon's *Symposium,* Socrates goes on to elaborate the way in which erotic relations function as modes of virtue production:

> But the greatest good that befalls the man who yearns (*oregomenō*) to make his darling pupil a good friend is the necessity of himself to practice virtue (*auton askein aretēn*). For to produce such a good companion one cannot be malicious, nor can he himself exhibit shamelessness and unwholesomeness and make his beloved (*eromenos*) reverent. (*Symposium* 8.27–28)

This passage suggests two important and related movements. First, Xenophon's character Socrates labels the proper, more valued erotics as those practices which lead to friendship, *philia.* As Foucault puts it, "The love of boys could not be morally honorable unless it comprised the elements that would form the basis of a transformation of this love into a definitive and socially valuable tie, that of *philia*" (1990: 225). Earlier in the speech, Socrates explains that those who seek *philia* have a greater investment in the partner's goodness (*Symposium* 8.25). This leads Socrates to the second important character of educative erotics:

if the *erastēs* wants to make the *eromenos* a friend, he must himself model virtuous behavior even as he expects it of the youth.[16]

As Dover points out, such passages suggest a kind of transferability of *aretē* from *erastēs* to *eromenos* (1978: 202). Some scholars even speculate that *aretē* was thought to be transmitted from *erastēs* to *eromenos* by way of the semen (Dover 1978: 202; Bethe 1907: 465–74; Devereux 1967: 80). The erotic relation therefore provided yet another mechanism through which *aretē* could be inculcated. Again, it is important to emphasize the nonlocatability of agency here; that the inculcation of *aretē* was thought to occur with ejaculation suggests that if anything receives agency it is the semen, the "carrier" of virtuosity. My point here is not to ascribe agency to fluid at all, but rather to suggest that just as ejaculation—an important humoral movement for the Greeks—is an effect of a particular intensity of encounter, so too is the related *phusiopoiesis*.

While ancient erotics, with its hierarchical requirements, defers the possibility of friendship, it also seeks to produce the bond of *philia* through an intensive connection that ultimately became a mode of transformation. Just as pain is not the necessary *telos* of the student-teacher relation, pleasure is not the ultimate goal of the male-male erotic dynamic. Having pain or pleasure as the aim would only re-inscribe subjectivity, reascribe agency. Rather, as Jean-Pierre Vernant puts it in his analysis of ancient *erōs,* "On the physical level, love between two beings consists in their engendering a third, different from each of them, which nonetheless prolongs them . . . Between two men, *erōs* tries to engender in the soul of the other beautiful discourses, beautiful virtues" (1990: 472–73). The "third" is the something other produced by phusiopoietic erotics, especially Platonic-Socratic erotics as detailed in *Phaedrus, Meno,* and the *Symposium.*

The love of wisdom—*philosophia*—could easily have been called *erōsophia,* as many sought out philosophical training with an intensity of passion understood better as *erōs.* This intensity could help explain why the sophists and their admirers are often referred to in Platonic dialogues as *erastai.* In the *Euthydemus,* for example, Socrates explains how upon the end of Dionysodorus' speech, the audience showed their approval for him and his sophist-comrade: "At that point there arose a great deal of laughter and loud applause from the pair's adorers (*erastai*), in wonder at their cleverness" (*Euthydemus* 276d). Similarly, Protagoras is linked to *erōs* when Socrates suggests that the group's coming to him demonstrates (*aphigmenoi*) an intense affinity (*hoti erastai*) for the old sophist (*Protagoras* 317c–d). In the opening of *Meno*, Socrates explains to the title character that Gorgias should be credited for "making the Thessalians enamored of wisdom (*erastas epi sophia*)" (*Meno* 70b).

The sophists, then, produced a dynamic of *erōsophia*, an intensive, zealous seeking out of wisdom, *sophia*. Still, the lines between *erōs* and *philia* were often indistinct, as Halperin, Winkler, and Zeitlin put it, "*erōs*, in Greek thinking, shades off into friendship and camaraderie, into that relationship of trust and reciprocity called *philia*" (Halperin, Winkler, and Zeitlin 1990: xvi). In relation to education, as Yun Lee Too points out, desire is what enables inquiry in the first place (2000: 64). The virtuous *erastēs* was nothing if not a teacher, bound to the possibility of transformation.

Phusiopoiesis thus occurred in a tangle of dynamics and forces. Desire emerges as an important component yoked to a variety of actions. The student's desire to transform constitutes submission to a training process, while the teacher's desire to provoke provides the necessary subjection. As I have tried to suggest, these forces of desire tended to follow painful and/or erotic trajectories, as pain and *philia* become two critical components of *phusiopoiesis*.

The transformative capacity of pain and erotic attachment effectively disrupts the boundaries of subjectivity by shaping and reshaping, by connecting and forging alliances among bodies, tools, cultural values, ethical principles, and futures. As such, pain and erotics emerge as *phusiopoietic* modes, arts of becoming that function as *allo*productions, in that they produce something other through their very combination. In other words, difference emerges through the connections forged in the painful and erotic acts observed in ancient educational dynamics.

The next two chapters will consider other phusiopoietic structures and mechanisms, examining more closely the space of the gymnasium and the ways in which the training dynamics there produced styles of existence through rhythmic habituation, imitation, and the repetitive movement of bodies.

Gymnasium I

The Space of Training

The opening of Plato's *Lysis* shows Socrates walking from the Academy to the Lyceum, two of Athens' three public gymnasia,[1] when he is intercepted by his friend Hippothales, who invites Socrates to venture in to join his circle of friends. The ensuing exchange, as narrated by the character Socrates, proceeds as follows:

> Where do you mean? I asked; and what is your company?
>
> Here, he said, showing me there, just opposite the wall, a sort of enclosure and a door standing open. We pass our time there (*diatribomen*), he went on; not only we ourselves, but others as well—a great many, and handsome.
>
> What is this place, and what do you do there (*kai tis ē diatribē*)?
>
> A wrestling school (*palaestra*), he said, of recent construction; and our pastime chiefly consists of discussions, in which we should be happy to let you have a share.
>
> That is very good of you, I said; and who does the teaching in there?
>
> Your own comrade, he replied, and supporter, Miccus. (*Lysis* 203b–4a; trans. adapted from Lamb)

Socrates has happened upon a private palaestra, common during his time in Athens, where young boys were sent to learn wrestling and other forms of gymnastics. Such venues were one of the markers of Greek cities, as the sophist from late antiquity Dio Chrysostom put it, "In each city of the Greeks there is a place set apart in which they go mad daily—the gymnasium" (*Oration* 32.44).

But more than that, Athenian gymnasia were also the site of philosophical discussions of the sort described here by Hippothales, in this case conducted by the sophist Miccus. Such discussions were understood as a kind of informal training, as they fostered the production and demonstration of skills important for public discourse, and the working through of particular cultural and philosophical topics, such as friendship in the example of *Lysis*. From Isidore of Seville's vantage in late antiquity: "A gymnasium is a general place for exercises. Yet at Athens it was the place where philosophy was learned and the pursuit of wisdom was 'exercised'" (*Etymologiae* 15.2.30). In Athens, then, the gymnasium combined the physical with the intellectual, and the sophists appear to have played major roles in this aspect of the gymnasium's history.

The Place of the Sophist

Evidence of sophistic activity in gymnasia and palaestrae is scattered throughout Greek writings. In *Panathenaicus,* Isocrates refers to the sophists' inhabiting of the Lyceum (18.33). Diogenes Laertius writes of Gorgias' student Antisthenes (444–365 BCE), who was the first to set up some sort of permanent school at Athens; he apparently located his school in the Cynosarges gymnasium and attracted a large group of students (*Lives* 6.1–13). In his treatise *Amatorius,* Plutarch mentions that his sons take philosophy in the wrestling school (2.749c). In the pseudo-Platonic dialogue *Eryxias* Prodicus is said to have been discoursing so loudly in the gymnasium that the gymnasiarch, the gymnasium overseer, had to ask him to keep the noise level down (397c–d). According to Plutarch, a public reading of Protagoras' *On the Gods* may well have taken place in the Lyceum (*Lives* 9.54). Sophists apparently infiltrated gymnasia in the beginning of the classical era and remained there until late antiquity.

To be sure, the sophists did not teach exclusively at gymnasia. Private houses also served as common meeting spots for sophistic exchanges. As R. E. Wycherley points out, "a Greek philosophical school was essentially a specialized extension of the Hellenic household" (1962: 155). It was common for citizens to play host to itinerant scholars, much like the scenarios found in Plato's dialogues. In the *Phaedrus,* for example, the dialogue's opening shows Phaedrus reporting to Socrates that he has just come from the house of Epicrates, where Phaedrus and Epicrates discoursed on the subject of *erōs*. Isocrates set up a school in his own house, as did Kallias (Wycherley 1962: 155–57). While Isocrates taught in a house, his place of teaching is said to have been located near the Lyceum,[2] and he surely spent some time at local athletic facilities, for he is said to have died in 338/37 in an Athenian palaestra owned by a man named Hippocrates (Kyle 1987: 144; Ps.-Plut., *Lives of the Ten Orators* 837e).

Other sophists wandered about town, often imparting their wisdom in the agora (marketplace). Xenophon tells how the sophist Euthydemus used a saddler's shop near the agora as a place for sharing his art of discourse (*Memorabilia* 4.2.1). In Plato's *Hippias Minor*, Socrates says to Hippias that he has heard him making a display of his wisdom "in the agora by the tables" (368b).

Most, if not all, sophists, though, passed through the city's gymnasia at some point. Plato and Aristotle thus followed the lead of the sophists when they set up their schools at the Academy and the Lyceum, respectively.

Apparently, all of Athens was swarming with sophists. These mobile teachers were particularly drawn to the spaces where they were likely to be most visible to potential clientele: the agora and the gymnasia both served this function. Visibility is then followed by a retreat to a more intimate space, be it a house, a saddle shop, a corner of a private palaestra, such as the one Socrates happens upon, or the "undressing room" of a public gymnasium.

For all practical purposes, the gymnasium, a sprawling space with numerous areas inhabited by young men, was an ideal place for sophists to cultivate a following. For one thing, as Susan Jarratt has observed, the sophists were the Athenian version of "public intellectuals" (1991b: 98), so it makes sense that they would visit the public gymnasia, since the sites were already an integral part of the daily practices of most free Athenian men. But perhaps more important, these locations were filled with youths seeking to cultivate a citizen *ēthos*. As Frederick Beck points out, "palaestrae and gymnasia were the only places of instruction frequented at all by boys in their middle and late teens" (1964: 131).

From this spatial intermingling of practices there emerged a specific syncretism between athletics and rhetoric, a particular crossover in pedagogical practices and learning styles, a crossover that contributed to the development of rhetoric as a bodily art: an art learned, practiced, and performed by and with the body as well as the mind.

As locations of physical training, the gymnasia were already phusiopoietic spaces where the production of "second nature" occurred: the gymnasia were recognized sites for the production of citizen subjects, and moreover, the production took place in a decidedly corporeal style. Furthermore, the gymnasium provided ample space and opportunities for sophistic training along with the gymnastic training already going on there. So the phusiopoietic economy produced and emerged out of educational spaces known as gymnasia and palaestrae.[3]

Such spaces functioned as disciplinary sites; and, as Michel Foucault writes, "discipline sometimes requires enclosures" (1979: 141). Whereas Foucault considers the productive, regulatory effects of particular institutional structures (a line of inquiry I will pursue here in terms of the uses and functions of ancient gymnasia), the ancient gymnasium, as we will see, was not so much an "enclosure," but it was nonetheless a dedicated space that functioned generatively to encourage and regulate activities and therefore subjectivities.

This chapter, then, will examine the space of the ancient Athenian gymnasium as a functional site of citizen production, part of the material complex that produced what Pierre Bourdieu calls *habitus,* "a system of lasting, transposable dispositions" (1978: 78) that produced body-mind complexes capable of metic, kairotic responses.

An examination of the layout of ancient gymnasia provides a way to imagine how bodies moved through and within the spaces, and a consideration of architectural changes over time provides a kind of material, longitudinal commentary on the way in which the gymnasium was in turn structured by emerging *habitus.*

Such a consideration folds back into the issues of virtue production considered in chapter 1, as the "stones of Athens" reveal the *polis*'s investment in forming particular body-mind complexes.[4] The uses and forms of ancient Athenian gymnasia were constituted by the emerging citizen *ēthos.* In other words, the disciplinary space of the gymnasium helps us imagine a particular articulation of formative practices and the ways in which these practices overlapped, repeated, and supported one another.

The available cultural information regarding Athenian gymnasia, such as archaeological findings, literary accounts, and depictions painted on pottery, enables us to piece together an idea of some of the architectural features and training apparatuses, as well as the movements and practices found in and around the gymnasium. Such information, tenuous and fragmented as it might be, still enables a consideration of the ways in which the ancient mind-body complex was shaped.

Uses of Ancient Gymnasia

The use of gymnasia and palaestrae for philosophical and rhetorical training (what Isocrates calls "gymnastics of the mind") began in the late fifth and fourth centuries and continued on through late antiquity.

The facilities themselves first emerged with the development of sports from informal games into organized athletics and the corollary need for a place to gather and exercise (Gardiner 1910: 467; Kyle 1987: 56). Prior to this development, athletic exercises likely took place in the Greek agora, the ancient gathering place *par excellence*. Archaeologists have uncovered remains of a running track with a starting gate in the Athenian Agora that dates to the fifth century (Thompson 1994: 22–23).

As Donald Kyle points out, early uses and functions of athletic training were multiple: "athletics possibly were related to funerary or initiatory rites, hero cults, festivals of unification, fertility or sacrifice, military influences and more" (1987: 10 n. 38). Similarly, athletic training facilities had religious and military affiliations. All three of Athens' public gymnasia are said to have originated as sanctuaries. The Lyceum, for example, was a sanctuary dedicated to Apollo the wolf slayer or wolf-god, as its name, *Lykeios,* indicates (Lynch 1972: 9–11). According to Diogenes Laertius, the namesake and patron of Plato's Academy is the hero Academus (3.7). Demosthenes puts it succinctly: "There were the three gymnasia at Athens. They were also sanctuaries (*hiera*): the Lyceum was dedicated to Apollo the Wolf-slayer, the Cynosarges to Herakles, and the Academy to the eponymous hero Academus" (Demosthenes, *Oration* 24.114).

Evidence of the military uses of gymnasia appears in archaeological fragments and literary works. The earliest classical reference to the Lyceum occurs in Aristophanes' *Peace* and refers to its military function, as the chorus describes how "for quite long enough we've been killing ourselves and worn ourselves out, wandering to the Lyceum and from the Lyceum, spear, shield, and all" (lines 353–57). Troops—both Athenian and foreign—gathered at the Academy and the Lyceum before expeditions. The troops of the Spartan general Pausanias and the Athenian Iphikrates both spent time training and dining in the Academy (Xen. *Hell.* 2.2.8; 6.5.49). Both sites offered wide spaces for such gathering and training, and the access to Athens and its water sources provided the amenities needed for military preparation (Kyle 1987: 77–79).

But the primary use of gymnasia, particularly in the Early Classical period, was to train the body in gymnastics. As is commonly known, *gymnasion* means, generally, "place where one goes to exercise naked," and so does not necessarily imply a fixed architectural structure. Early gymnasia were rudimentary in that they consisted simply of *dromoi,* long pathlike racetracks situated in groves. In the Archaic era, according to Kyle (1987), gymnasia were demarcated by walled gardens with *dromoi* and palaestrae, open-air sites for wrestling exercises (*palaiō* means to wrestle). Such sites were usually situated on the outskirts of a city in a spot with ample shade and a stream. This was certainly true of the Academy, the Lyceum, and the Cynosarges, the three public gymnasia of Athens (Gardiner 1910: 468). The late fifth, fourth, and third centuries saw the emergence of gymnasia as permanent architectural structures, with colonnaded walkways (called *peripatoi*) and hot baths, which evolved into the more elaborate Roman bath complexes of late antiquity.[5]

While some palaestrae were privately owned, the public had access to several. As pseudo-Xenophon writes in *Constitution of the Athenians,* "the *dēmos* have built for their own use many wrestling areas, undressing rooms, and baths. The general populace (*ochlos*) has more enjoyment of these things than the few (*oligoi*)" (2.10). Here, pseudo-Xenophon reveals details about the use of gymnasia by more than just elite citizens. In many ways, the gymnasium was a democratic, collective space; Delormé points out that the gymnasium served the same function for the boys and young men of Athens as the agora did for the adult citizens (1960: 316).

In other words, in addition to its athletic training function, the gymnasium was a place to gather, to socialize, to develop and share ideas. There were sociopolitical boundaries, however, as slaves were prevented by law from use of the gymnasia (Aeschines, *Against Timarchus* 1.138), and there is no evidence that women frequented the facilities. Furthermore, Plutarch suggests that *nothoi*—those from outside Athens, or those with only one Athenian parent—frequented only Cynosarges (*Lives.* 1.3).[6]

In effect, then, the gymnasium functioned as a gathering place for

Athenian male citizens and for citizens-in-training. The gathering function is underscored by the following inscription from the first century BCE, which relates to the Lyceum and reads

Dionysios the son of Dionysodoros
[Of the Kekropid tribe,] overseer
Of the Lyceum [dedicated this] to Apollo
In the gymnasiarchy of Kallikratides
The upholder of the gathering (*sundromou*)
(Travlos 1980: 347; trans. Walker)

Here the dedicatory inscription contains all the pertinent information about its dedicator, and more important for our purposes, it invokes the gymnasiarch as the person in charge of maintaining the "gathering," *sundromos,* a word invoking a convergence of a certain intensity, as it may even be translated "muscle contraction." Here it is Kallikrates who presided over the throng; the period of his term, as well as that of other gymniarchs, was known as a "gymniarchy."

Given the concentrated gathering facilitated by the gymnasium, it is no surprise that Athenian leaders took a great deal of interest in the operations of gymnastic facilities. Leaders in the Classical period did much to develop and maintain the structures. Pericles is thought to have directed public resources toward the construction and development of the Lyceum (Kyle 1987: 101; Lynch 1972: 15–16), and Lycurgus is credited with renovating that gymnasium in the fourth century (Lynch 1972: 15–16; Delormé 1960: 42). Themistocles is thought to have helped establish the Cynosarges, while his rival, the politician Kimon, was known to have renovated the athletic facilities at the Academy during his reign (Kyle 1987: 71, 100).

The gymnasiarch, the person in charge of the gymnasium's daily operations and provisions, was considered a public official (Forbes 1945: 33). The gymnasium was also the focus of specific legislation. Demosthenes invokes an Athenian law making theft of property from the Lyceum, the Academy, or the Cynosarges punishable by death (*Against Timocrates* 24.114), while Aeschines, Demosthenes' rival, cites laws prohibiting the opening of the palaestra before sunrise and mandating its closing before sunset (*Against Timarchus* 10).[7]

Even though all three of Athens' public gymnasia lay outside the city walls, they were still easily accessible and were considered a major element of city life, a kind of extension of the city; indeed, the gymnasium was viewed across Greece as one of the legitimating marks of a *polis,* as indicated by Pausanias' negative assessment of Panopoeus, "a city of the Phocians, if one can give the name of city to those that possess no government offices, no gymnasium, no theater, no agora, no water conducted to a fountain" (10.4.1). For Pausanias, loci for gathering, such as the gymnasium, the theater, and the agora, were as necessary to city life as government and running water.

But more than that, the gymnasium functioned as the primary locus for citizen production; gymnasia were just as integral to the city's future as to its present, and were thus imbued with purposive political interest. It was in the gymnasia that most of Athens' future leaders were trained, at least to some degree. Gymnasia were therefore intimately connected with the life of the *polis;* indeed, they functioned as extensions of it— both geographically and temporally.

Spatial Distribution

The pseudo-Xenophon passage cited above, in addition to remarking on who used the public gymnasia, also gives some indication of the kinds and number of rooms in the Classical gymnasium, as he mentions wrestling areas, undressing rooms, and baths.

The most thorough description of the Classical Greek gymnasium's architectural structure is found in the work of the Roman architect Vitruvius. Although Vitruvius wrote from the vantage point of late antiquity, he was nonetheless an expert in Greek architecture with a particular interest in houses, temples, theaters, and athletic facilities. Vitruvius confirms and greatly elaborates the Xenophonic description of gymnasia, and as Harold Harris suggests, the Academy and the Lyceum may have been configured in the gymnasium pattern he describes (1966: 146). Stephen Glass, in a lengthy analysis of early gymnasium structures, observes that the literary accounts of fifth- and fourth-century palaestra and gymnasia hold "faint glimmerings of the basic structure which Vitruvius proposes" (1967: 68).

Vitruvius' account of the architectural features of the Greek gymnasium enables commentary on the distribution of bodies in space and the movement between various activities at the site. Figure 5.1 features a diagram of a palaestra according to Vitruvius' detailed directions for constructing an athletic facility based on the Greek model, excerpted below.

In the three colonnades construct roomy recesses (A) with seats in them, where philosophers, rhetoricians, and others who delight in learning may sit and discourse. In the double colonnade let the rooms be arranged thus: the young men's hall (B) in the middle; this is a very spacious recess (*exedra*) with seats in it, and it should be one-third longer than it is broad. At the right, the bag room [a room equipped with punching bags] (C); then next, the dust room [where athletes dusted themselves in preparation for training or competition] (D); beyond the dust room, at the corner of the colonnade, the cold washing room (E), which the Greeks call *loutron*. At the left of the young men's hall is the anointing room (F); then, next to the anointing room, the cold bath room (G), and beyond that a passage into the furnace room (H) at the corner of the colonnade. Next, but inside and on a line with the cold bath room, put the vaulted sweating bath (I), its length twice its breadth, and having at the ends on one side a Laconicum (K), proportioned in the same manner as above described, and opposite the Laconicum the warm washing room (L).

Inside a palaestra, the peristyle ought to be laid out as described above. But on the outside, let the three colonnades be arranged, one as you leave the peristyle and two at the right and left, with running-tracks in them. That one of them which faces the north should be a double colonnade of very ample breadth, while the other should be single, and so constructed that on the sides next to the walls and the side along the columns it may have edges, serving as paths, of not less than ten feet, with the space between them sunken, so that steps are necessary in going down from the edges a foot and a half to the plane, which plane should not be less than twelve feet wide. Thus people walking around on the edges will not be interfered with by the anointed who are exercising. (Vitruvius, *de Arch.* 5.11.2–3; trans. Morgan)

Vitruvius' rendering of the ancient gymnasium aligns well with archaeological excavations of Greek gymnasium sites, especially those diagrammed by Delormé, whose extensive study *Gymnasion* (1960) is still the foremost authority on ancient gymnasia. Figure 5.2 shows Delormé's plan of the gymnasium in the sanctuary of Apollo on the island of Delos. In the middle is the wrestling area, which is surrounded by rooms similar to those described by Vitruvius.

Starting with the large western room (G), the *apodyterion* (undressing room), and moving clockwise, we have the washing room (E), a second undressing room (D), a long *exedra* (C), a *sphairistra*, or a ball-playing room (B). The gymnasium at Epidaurus (not pictured) aligns with Vitruvius' description and is almost identical to the gymnasium at Olympia (figure 5.3), which may have provided the model for Vitruvius' description and might have been modeled on Athenian gymnasia. The gymnasium at Delphi (figure 5.4) differs slightly because it is apparently crafted to complement the difficult landscape on the steep slope of Mount Parnassus.

All these sites, however, feature the common elements of ancient gymnasia: a square, open wrestling area and functional rooms in the middle for dressing, oiling, and dusting. With the exception of the gymnasium at Delphi, which was constructed earlier, in the fourth century BCE, the gymnasia illustrated here are from the Hellenistic period. While likely more elaborate than Early Classical gymnasia structures, of which virtually no evidence remains, they were most probably modeled on the structures at Athens, which at the very least had one or two spacious rooms for changing and bathing in addition to the large wrestling area.

The Academy gymnasium can also be traced to the Early Classical period; it features a design somewhat similar to that described by Vitruvius. Figure 5.5 shows John Travlos' restored plan of this site (1980), with the darker black areas indicating the extant remains. According to Travlos, the peristyle (square center) dates to the second half of the 4th century BCE, after Plato established his school at the Academy in 388 (1980: 43). The restored plan shows a large rectangular area with a smaller palaestra in the middle and an oblong area to the north for bathing facilities. While the excavated gymnasium dates to the end of the Hellenistic period, the area itself as a site for gathering dates back to the 6th century BCE, when it was enclosed by a wall, according to the Suida (Travlos 1980: 42). The excavated northernmost rectangular peristyle dates to the 4th century (43). Once again, in line with Vitruvius' description, the wrestling area is surrounded by the typical colonnades on three sides, with the various rooms for dressing and bathing on the fourth.

Just as valuable as his description of the gymnasium's structure is Vitruvius' explicit rationalization for its spatial organization. Most notable, for the purposes of this study at least, is his call for wide spaces to allow for the variety of activities in the gymnasium—thanks to the width of

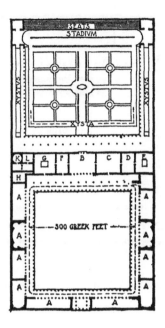

FIGURE 5.1
Plan of gymnasium based on Vitruvius' description.
From Morgan 1960: 161.

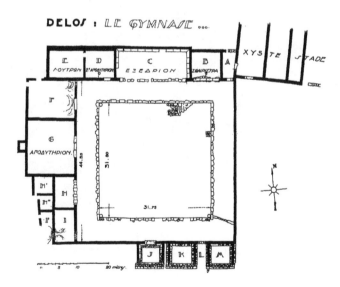

FIGURE 5.2
Plan of the gymnasium at Delos. From Delormé 1960: fig. 36, pl. xix.

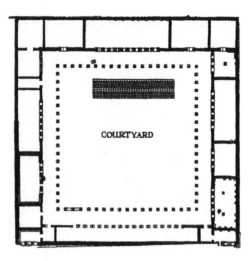

FIGURE 5.3

Plan of the gymnasium at Olympia. From Delormé 1960: fig. 21, pl. xii.

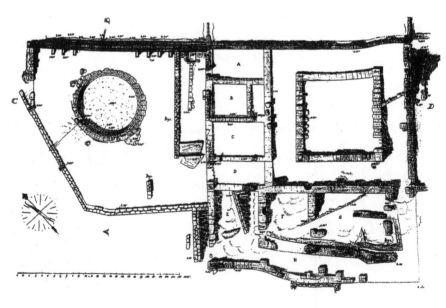

FIGURE 5.4

Plan of the gymnasium at Delphi. From Delormé 1960: fig. 12, pl. vi.

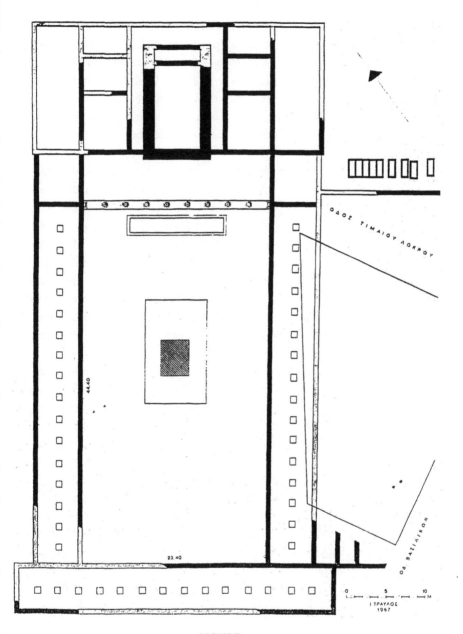

FIGURE 5.5
Plan of the Academy in Athens. From Travlos 1980: fig. 59.

the colonnades, philosophers and rhetoricians walking around discussing matters in the style of Aristotle's peripatetic school were less likely to collide with runners or javelin throwers practicing their form (Vitruvius, *de Arch.* 5.11.4). Still, the kinetic activities likely overlapped with one another in some sense, as youths moved from lectures and practice in rhetoric and philosophy with the sophists to learning and practicing wrestling maneuvers under the watchful eyes and hovering fork of the *paidotribēs*.

The colonnades, the *exedrae,* the undressing room, and the groves and walks, in the case of the Academy and the Lyceum,[8] were the areas in the gymnasium where philosophers and sophists would gather with youths for rhetorical and philosophical training. These areas, as indicated by the various plans described above, are part of the rhythmic flow of traffic through the facility. The open-air colonnades follow the circumference of the wrestling area; the undressing room—the space where athletes go to prepare for training and where they return when the day's exercises are complete—and the *exedrae,* the large lecture areas, by Vitruvius' description, are all situated around the palaestra proper.

The space itself, insofar as it provides ample room for and distributes the activities, allows for several educational practices to take place at once. Young boys would move deliberately from one activity to another, as Diogenes Laertius makes clear in his description of Aristotle in the Lyceum, "where he would walk up and down discussing philosophy with his pupils until it was time [for them] to rub themselves with oil" (5.2). In Plato's *Theatetus* we see another example of the easy movement between gymnastic and philosophical endeavors when Theodorus and Socrates spot Theatetus among his friends. Theodorus points him out as "the middle one of those who are approaching now. He and those friends of his were anointing themselves in the outer course (*hexō dromō*), and now they seem to me to be coming here" (144c; translation mine). Indeed, Theatetus approaches—perhaps even still pink-faced and sweaty from exercising—and a hearty discussion of knowledge and *technē* ensues.

It is precisely in the spaces among the areas where agonistic athletic training was occurring that instances of early training in rhetoric and philosophy took place—in the gymnasium's spacious colonnades and *exedrae,* as well as in the undressing area, a functional space we will now examine more closely.

The Un-Dressing Room

Integral to athletic training were the practices of preparation, most of which took place in the *apodyterion,* literally the "un-dressing room," or the stripping location.

Figures 5.6 and 5.7 show two sides of an early-fifth-century red-figure kylix, both of which depict activities in the *apodyterion.* On the wall to the right in both scenes, we see a discus sling (on side B the discus is in its place), and each scene shows two oil flasks, indispensable artifacts in the ancient gymnasium. Oiling was the central part of the preparation ritual, as all athletes covered their bodies with olive oil prior to competition or training. This practice was mostly a hygienic measure, as oil served to keep dirt, sand, and dust out of the pores (Harris 1966: 102). A tradition of massaging likely emerged from the oil-rubbing as well. For wrestlers, oil made gripping difficult, so they dusted themselves with a fine powder before competing.

On side B (fig. 5.7) the oil flasks are accompanied by strigils, long, curved, dull-edged bronze instruments used to scrape oil and powder off the body when the athletes were finished exercising. Side A (fig. 5.6) shows one athlete scraping himself with a strigil (the second figure from the left). Side A also features a dead hare hanging on the wall or from the ceiling. Gardiner speculates that one of the youths has just caught the hare, has brought it as a gift to the trainer, or has just received it as a prize (1910: 477).

On side B (fig. 5.7), a naked man (far left) leans on his stick next to a stool with a folded mantle on it (a long piece of material worn draped around the shoulders). To the right of the stool is a youth holding jumping weights (*haltereis*) in each hand. The weights were used for training in strength and balance while practicing the long jump. Two more figures engage in some kind of exchange over an item held in the man's outstretched hand.

Athletes often received assistance in preparation from *aleiptes,* young attendants who worked for palaestra and gymnasium owners. Figures 5.8 and 5.9 show both sides of an Archaic krater and feature four *aleipteis.* In figure 5.8, the kneeling attendant on the left examines (or massages) the youth's left foot. The attendant on the far right stands by waiting to take an athlete's mantle. In the center, an athlete pours oil into his left hand. The athletes are all preparing for exercise, and as the vase scene attests, preparations were somewhat elaborate.

Figure 5.9 shows similar practices; the youth at left-center holds a discus in his raised arms while a second youth points at the discus-bearer's genitals. The youth on the left is looking down at his own genitals, which are stretched out in his left hand. A nearby attendant looks on.

As the vase scenes suggest, the *apodyterion* was the site for more than just preparation for training. The preparation practices themselves took up a good deal of time and created opportunities for leisurely exchanges and relaxation time, as suggested by the figures who lean on sticks and stand around chatting. Figures 5.8 and 5.9 indicate that the practices in the *apodyterion* were often erotically charged, as youths interacted in close proximity, with and without clothing, rubbing oil on and massaging each other, and bathing together. The *apodyterion* became a primary gathering spot, a locus for all kinds of exchanges inside gymnasia and palaestrae. The youths are making themselves ready for the phusiopoietic transformation delineated in chapter 4.

Plato's *Lysis* amplifies the gathering function of the *apodyterion*, as Socrates follows Hippothales' urgings and ventures inside the palaestra to engage with the sophists there, as well as to meet the object of Hippothales' desire, for whom the dialogue is named (204b–e). As the character Socrates describes it, some kind of sacrifice had taken place in the facility just prior to his arrival (206e). In postsacrificial form, well-dressed youths were playing together in the outdoor court, but others were found in the *apodyterion* playing a game with knucklebones, with observers gathered around.

As Socrates narrates it, "as for us, we went and sat apart on the opposite side—for it was quiet there—and started some talk among ourselves" (*Lysis* 207a). The undressing area must have been rather large for Socrates and his friends to find a quiet corner. Soon, though, Lysis and some of the other youths watching the game, curious about the discussion starting on the other side of the room, wander over to join Socrates' group. The rest of the dialogue, a discussion of friendship, takes place entirely in the undressing room, apparently a common spot for sophistic exchanges.

The *Euthydemus*, an account of another series of sophistic exchanges, this time set in the Lyceum, also takes place in the *apodyterion* (272e). In this dialogue, Socrates' exchange takes place with Euthydemus and Dionysodorus, two brothers well known for their skill in the pankration (a combination of wrestling and boxing) as well as their compe-

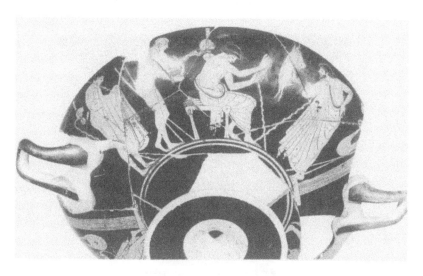

FIGURE 5.6

Scene from the *apodyterion,* from an Athenian red-figure kylix: Thorvaldsens
Museum H612, side A. © Thorvaldsens Museum, Copenhagen.

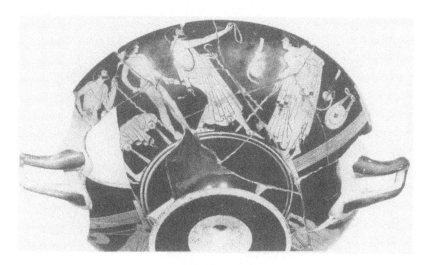

FIGURE 5.7

Scene from the *apodyterion,* from an Athenian red-figure kylix: Thorvaldsens
Museum H612, side B. © Thorvaldsens Museum, Copenhagen.

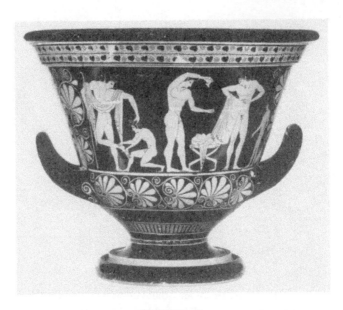

FIGURE 5.8
Scene showing preparations for training, from an Athenian red-figure krater:
Berlin Antikenmuseen F2180, side A. © Berlin Antikenmuseen.

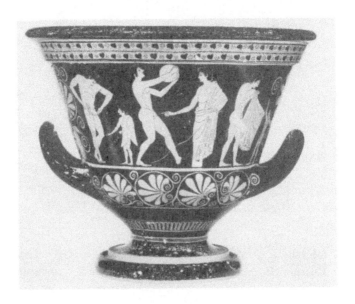

FIGURE 5.9
Scene showing preparations for training, from an Athenian red-figure krater:
Berlin Antikenmuseen F2180, side B. © Berlin Antikenmuseen.

tence in the law courts. The brothers inform Socrates that they are at the Lyceum to exhibit and explain their art to anyone who wishes to learn it (274b).[9]

Apparently those wishing to learn from the sophists were many. As Crito recalls in the opening of the dialogue, there was such a crowd around Socrates and the sophists in the undressing room that day that he could barely hear or see what was going on, so he asks, "Who was it, Socrates, that you were talking with yesterday at the Lyceum? Why, there was such a crowd standing about you that when I came up in the hope of listening I could hear nothing distinctly: still, by craning over I got a glimpse" (*Euthydemus* 271A; trans. Lamb).

When Socrates tells of the brothers' entry, he describes their movement in a throng: "So I sat down again, and after a little while these two persons entered—Euthydemus and Dionysodorus—and, accompanying them, quite a number, as it seemed to me, of their pupils; the two men came in and began walking along inside the cloister (*dromō*)" (*Euthydemus* 272e–73a; trans. Lamb). As Lamb notes, the *dromos* encompassed the open court in the center and could be accessed through the undressing room (1932: 385 n. 3).

These passages, along with the *apodyterion* scenes in *Lysis* and on the vases discussed above, point to a critical function of the undressing room's space: its facilitation of gathering. In both *Theatetus* and *Lysis*, the title characters are introduced as approaching with a group of friends, ostensibly coming from anointing or competing, but most certainly as part of a larger group, much like that recounted by Socrates in *Euthydemus*.

The undressing room, with its expansive space and time-consuming, almost laconic preparatory practices, facilitated crowd formation. The ancient gymnasium thus encouraged gathering, association with others —with other citizens in training, with *paidotribeis*, with sophists and philosophers, with lovers. No doubt the formation of crowds around sophists was part of their seduction. The spaces the sophists inhabited, already scenes of crowd formation, certainly helped feed the seductive effect of their teachings.

Of course such crowds formed and dispersed, as youths moved among the many activities that took place in the *apodyterion*—the usual preparatory and postexercise activities of oiling, dusting, scraping, and bathing—along with more leisurely activities such as massaging and game-playing. The *apodyterion*, already infused with ritualistic preparation, desire, and the energy anticipating self-transformation, served as the ideal spot for intellectual intercourse. The undressing room, as part of the youth's daily cycle of gathering and dispersing, provided an integral structure for the Athenian *habitus.*

The strategic infiltration of sophistic activity into this regularly inhabited space thus allowed for the production of new habits and practices. That is to say, when encountering sophists and philosophers daily at regular intervals, the youths were no doubt subject—consciously or not—to their teachings. Sophistic training became a part of the regular cycle of education at athletic facilities, a characteristic feature of bodily training for rising citizens.

The inculcation of such knowledge in a crowd heightens the embodied nature of such learning, as the space of the ancient gymnasium emerged as part of a network of forces—other youths, bathing and massaging, sophists, the practice of oiling, philosophers, strigils, the gathering and dispersal of crowds. This network of objects, people, and practices and their attendant sounds and smells comprised a distinctive material setting for a highly textured, bodily pedagogy. The situating of rhetorical training temporally and spatially in the midst of athletic training likely produced a set of linked habits—the habits of discursive moves and wrestling moves, the habits of competing, pushing, developing, responding—linked if not in the mind, then certainly in the body.

While the next chapter will examine the sophistic style of phusiopoietic habit production more closely, I first want to briefly examine the way in which the crowding tendencies and habituated practices produced evolutionary effects on the gymnasium, and by extension, the educational practices there.

Restructuring Structures

The infiltration of gymnasia and palaestrae by sophists and philosophers effectively changed the facilities' structures over time. The most notable change, aside from the broadening of colonnades and the addition of benches described by Vitruvius, was the development of libraries within gymnasia. Aristotle, who followed the sophists' and Plato's lead in setting up a school at a public gymnasium, was the first to make a systematic and substantial collection of books for his school (Lynch 1972: 97; Strabo, *Geographies* 13.1.54). Athenaeus lists Aristotle's as one of the important ancient libraries (*Deipnosophistai* 1.3a). Aristotle's collection may well have exceeded the space at the Lyceum; Lynch cites this as a possible reason for the establishment of a nearby private garden when his successor, Theophrastus, took over the school (Lynch 1972: 83–85).

After the Classical period, during which *paidotribai*, sophists, and philosophers seemed to have comfortably inhabited the space oᵢ the gymnasium together, rhetorical and philosophical activity began to supersede athletic activity, though this transition took at least a century (Gardiner 1967: 149). The early sophists had left their mark, as their infiltration helped reconfigure not only educational practices, but also the very space of the gymnasium. As Delormé characterizes these later periods, it was "rhétorique avant tout," rhetoric before everything (1960: 331).

The construction of the first public gymnasium inside Athens' walls, while it did not happen until the Hellenistic age, provides some insight into such reconfiguration. Established by Ptolemy Philadelphus in the mid-third century BCE, the Ptolemaion served as a locus for ephebic (adolescent) education.

The most notable feature of this building, at least for this study's purposes, is its possession of a library, formed and subsidized by its students and lecturers. Figure 5.10 shows the Gymnasium of Ptolomy plan as restored by Travlos (1980). On the eastern side (bottom of figure) is the oblong hall, which originally had twelve marble structures set in the floor to support wooden tables or desks; this was likely the location of the building's library (Travlos 1980: 233). Also noteworthy in this gymnasium as compared to the earlier structures is the expansion of the colonnades and lecture halls. The wrestling area, the square room to the southwest, which had previously been the largest, most central part of the gymnasium, was by this time dwarfed in comparison to the sprawling stoa and walkways.

The changing morphology of the ancient gymnasium signals larger transformations in educational practices. For instance, the incorporation of broader colonnades and larger lecture halls in some of the gymnasium structures discussed above appears to be a way of accommodating the crowds attracted by sophists.

While during the Classical period the practices of athletic and rhetorical training seemed to have comfortably inhabited the same space as joint arts of existence, the shared space began to pose more of a prob-

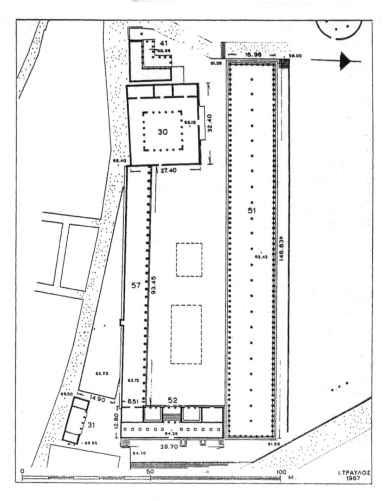

FIGURE 5.10
Plan of the Gymnasium of Ptolemy. From Travlos 1980: fig. 303.

lem as bodily training began to be disparaged. Cicero himself depicts objections to the spatial convergence. As his character Crassus puts it:

> It is my belief that even the Greeks themselves devised their exercise-ground, benches and colonnades for purposes of physical training and enjoyment, not for dialectic. For not only were there gymnastic schools introduced ages before the philosophers began to chatter therein, but even in the present day, although the sages

may be in occupation of all the gymnastic schools, yet their audiences prefer to listen to the discus rather than to the Master, and the moment its clink is heard, they all desert the lecturer, in the middle of an oration upon the most sublime and weighty topics, in order to anoint themselves for athletic exercise. (*de Oratore* 2.5.21; trans. Sutton and Rackham)

Here, Crassus describes tension between the development of the mind and the development of the body, a tension still left over in his time that emerged most palpably toward the end of the Classical period and into the Hellenistic age, as athletics became more specialized, and, as a result, gymnastics became cordoned off—spatially and practically—from the overall curriculum.

The ambivalent account given by Crassus here contains tacit assumptions about the way athletic training "detracted" from more "noble" pursuits in the lectures. What Crassus' account has forgotten, however, is the way in which training in rhetoric and philosophy during the Classical period was intimately bound up with—and even, to some extent, drew its educational methods from—athletic training.

The next chapter will deal more precisely with the overlapping of training practices—the specific ways in which habits were produced in the gymnasium. But these practices need to be considered in conjunction with—indeed, as constituted by—the space of the gymnasium. As this chapter has shown, the broad colonnades and large divisions of space facilitated fluid group movement between activities, allowing sophists to lecture and teach forms of thought in the undressing room, in the spaces and times between gymnastic training.

The spatial confluence helps clarify why Isocrates and Plato write of these pedagogical situations in terms of gymnastics. That is, the connections between the two arts emerged from daily habitual movement between athletic and rhetorical activities. While anointing and dusting his body, a young Athenian citizen in training might be seduced by a sophistic discourse on friendship, love, or the art of speaking well. Likewise, while listening to such lectures he could be called to anoint himself and prepare for a grapple in the wrestling room. The discursive movements, bound as they were with bodily training, emerged as an art of becoming that overlapped with and repeated the very movements and methods in gymnastic training.

The connections between rhetorical and athletic training, as will be demonstrated more fully in the next chapter, were therefore bodily, methodological, and habitual. Such connections were fostered by the traffic in the gymnasium, and facilitated by the hospitable reception of the sophists and the spatial distribution of bodies.

❉ 6 ❉

Gymnasium II

The Bodily Rhythms of Habit

A number of vase paintings illustrate Archaic school scenes that offer a glimpse of ancient training practices. Figure 6.1, side A of a kylix from 480 BCE, shows two lessons occurring simultaneously. The first, on the left, features a lyre lesson with the bearded teacher sitting on the left facing the student; the second shows the teacher with an inscribed scroll that reads "Muse to me . . . I begin to sing of wide-flowing Scamander," suggesting the two are in the midst of a recitation session (Havelock 1986: 203).

Figure 6.2, side B of the same kylix, shows first, on the left, a singing lesson with the teacher playing a double *aulos* (a pipelike reed instrument common to the period)[1] as accompaniment. Next to the singing lesson is a writing lesson; the teacher, seated on a cushioned stool, holds a writing tablet on his lap and a stylus in his raised right hand.

The interior of the kylix (not shown here) is quite telling in terms of the artifact's context: it features a naked youth bending to untie his sandal. The youth's staff lies on the *louterion* (washbasin) behind him, and his clothing (a mantle) is draped over a nearby stool. A sponge and an oil flask hang above the stool. This scene contains enough symbolic markers to connect the school scenes to the gymnasium, for it is set in a gymnasium washing room and depicts an athlete either before or after some kind of gymnastic exercises.

Figure 6.3 offers a glimpse of athletes such as the one mentioned above from the interior of the kylix; this time, they are well oiled, completely naked, and practicing in a gymnasium. Here we see pentathletes rehearsing the movements of javelin and discus throwing. A third ath-

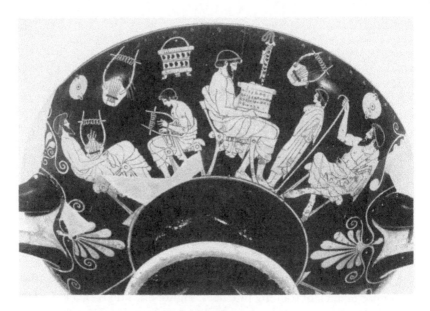

FIGURE 6.1
School scene depicted on an Athenian red-figure kylix: Berlin
Antikenmuseen F2285, side A. © Berlin Antikenmuseen.

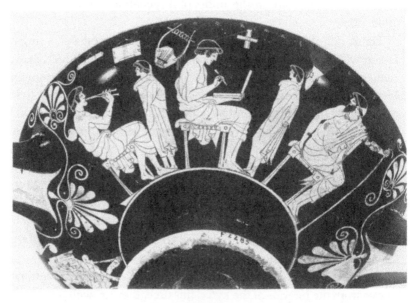

FIGURE 6.2
School scene depicted on an Athenian red-figure kylix: Berlin
Antikenmuseen F2285, side B. © Berlin Antikenmuseen.

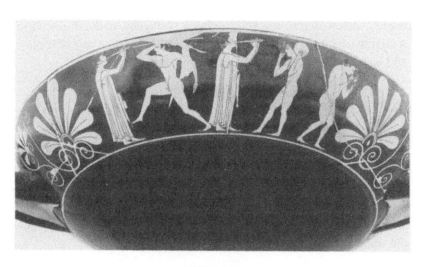

FIGURE 6.3
Scene showing pentathletes and *aulos*-players in the palaestra, from an
Athenian red-figure kylix: Berlin Antikenmuseen F2262, side A.
© Berlin Antikenmuseen.

lete, to the far right, is shadowboxing, an age-old practice wherein the
boxer-in-training jabs and practices footwork without an opponent (but
for his "shadow"). What's more, the cup featured here shows the athletes interspersed with *aulos*-players, instruments strapped to their chin
and heads lifted, indicating they are in the act of playing their pipes.

Noteworthy in these scenes is the recurring presence of musicians—
aulos- and lyre-players—which points to the intermingling of music
with other forms of training. As such, the vases suggest yet another element common to athletic and rhetorical training and thus worthy of
consideration here: the sounds of the Greek gymnasium.

While the last chapter considered the intermingling of practices in
the space of the gymnasium, this chapter will extend that exploration
while continuing the inquiry into *phusiopoiesis*, by examining more
closely the practices through which habits were cultivated in this important space. As this chapter will suggest, rhetorical training derived
from athletics and early education a style of training grounded in imitation and based on what I'm calling the three Rs of sophistic pedagogy—
rhythm, repetition, and response.

Such training took place in a decidedly corporeal style. This chapter will thus move to a consideration, through the examples of Demos-

thenes' rhetorical training and Isocrates' pedagogy, of the implications such practices hold for rhetoric as a performing practice, as a discipline, and as a bodily art.[2] But first, let's begin with a rhythm.

A Rhythmic Invasion

Each palaestra had at least one *aulos*-player associated with it. It was the *aulos*-player's job to set the rhythm for all gymnastic exercises, including the general warmup activities (as shown in fig. 6.3) and the focused practice of specific bodily movement. To the rhythm of the music, javelin throwers, wrestlers, boxers (fig. 6.4), jumpers (fig. 6.5), and other athletes would rehearse fundamental movements, be they throwing form, an approach or hold, or jab steps.

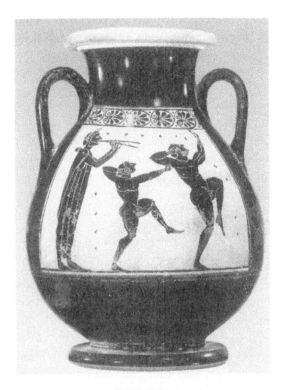

FIGURE 6.4
Scene showing boxers and *aulos*-player, from an Athenian
red-figure hydria: Metropolitan Museum of Art 49.11.1, side B.
© The Metropolitan Museum of Art, New York, Rodgers Fund, 1949.

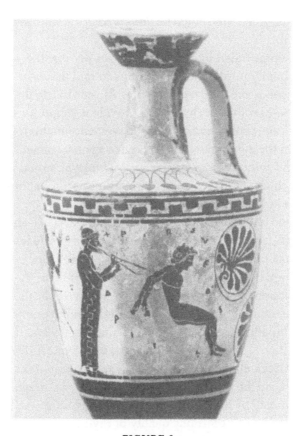

FIGURE 6.5

Scene showing jumper and *aulos*-player from an Athenian red-figure
lekythos: Metropolitan Museum of Art 08.258.30, side A.
© The Metropolitan Museum of Art, New York, Rodgers Fund, 1908.

It appears that *aulos*-players were almost as omnipresent as *paidotribai,* suggesting that music's role in bodily shaping was just as critical as
the instructor himself—indeed, I will argue that music was instructive
in its own way.

Given the proximity of athletic and rhetorical training, as well as the
noisiness of *auloi*—their shrill sounds approximate those produced by
modern-day bagpipes—it is also likely that music flowed into recita-
tions and sophistic lectures, producing an awareness of—perhaps facilitating—the rhythmic, tonic quality of speeches. As Kenneth J. Freeman points out, the *aulos* did not merely provide background noise, but
rather it played an integral role in training, as the instrument was used

"in order that good time might be preserved in the various movements" (1969: 128).

If, as demonstrated in chapter 4, we can say that the *paidotribēs* focused on bodily position, then we can add that the *aulos*-player regulated the speeds and intervals of motion. Music's role in the gymnasium then was to introduce a rhythm, to provide a tempo for the practice, regulation, and production of bodily movements. In this regard, the use of music in the gymnasium invoked once again a connection between athletic and military practices, as an *aulos*-player would also accompany marching soldiers, providing rhythmic accompaniment to keep their steps in time (Landels 1998: 8).

This kind of continuous rhythm, with its cyclical and repetitive movements, set the stage for—indeed, helped produce—two of the components of habit formation this chapter will examine: repetition and imitation. Put simply, music established a rhythm through the cyclical repetition of patterns, and this rhythm was replicated in the bodily movements of those in training. As Mark Griffith points out, the use of music "to align corporal, emotional, and intellectual impulses into a 'harmonious' set of 'habits' (*ethē* or *hexis*), is typical of Archaic and Classical Greek attitudes" (2001: 44). As such, music was an important carryover from the types of fifth-century educational practices depicted at the beginning of this chapter. For the ancients, music facilitated training through the habit-forming quality of rhythm.

As with most topics, Aristotle was the first to delineate the logic behind music in education.[3] For Aristotle, the intrinsic qualities of certain rhythms and modes were intractably connected to their effects on a person, so that some music proves useful for relaxation, some for education, some for pleasure, and some for catharsis (*Politics* 8.5.4–7). After parsing out the various effects of music, Aristotle moves to what is, at least for Aristotle, the more interesting line of inquiry—the way in which music works directly on character (*ēthos*) and soul (*psychē*):

> But it is evident that a certain quality is produced, both by many other kinds of music and not least by the melodies of Olympus; for these admittedly make our souls inspired, and inspiration is an affection of the soul's character (*enthusiasmos tou peri tēn psychēn ēthous pathos estin*). And besides, everybody, when listening to imitations (*mimēseōn*) enters into a state of sympathy, even apart from the rhythms and tunes themselves. (*Politics* 8.5.5–6)

For Aristotle, the aurality of music differs from other mimetic arts in that it more powerfully conveys *ēthos* than those arts depending on other senses for perception. He writes that "other objects of sensation contain no representation of character, for example, the objects of touch and taste" (*Politics* 8.5.7). He then offers a long parenthetical comment on visual art, where he says such works "are not representations of character but rather the forms and colors produced are mere indications of character" (*Politics* 8.5.8). By contrast, pieces of music "actually contain in themselves imitations of character" (*mimēmata tōn ēthōn*). Aristotle explicitly discusses different kinds of rhythms in terms of *possessing* (*echousi*) more stable (*stasimōteron*) or mobile (*kinētikon*) character (1340b9). In other words, music, with its sonorous, seductive movements, most closely approximates human *ēthos*, and the likeness produces a bond of sorts, as Aristotle writes, "we seem to have a certain kinship (*suggeneia*) with tunes and rhythms" (*Politics* 8.5.9).

Aristotle draws his conceptions of musical *ēthos* from the sophist Damon, a legendary music teacher who studied with the sophist Prodicus. According to a Damonian fragment, "Song and dance necessarily arise when the soul is in some way moved; liberal and beautiful songs and dances create a similar soul, and the reverse kind create (*poiousi*) a reverse kind of soul" (DK 37 B6).[4] Hence, for Damon, music and its attendant practices of song and dance are productive arts; they directly produce (*poiousi*) particular kinds of souls. Along the same lines, Plato's Socrates contends that "rhythm and harmonies have the greatest influence on the soul; they penetrate into its inmost regions and there hold fast (*haptetai*)" (*Republic* 401d). The soul-gripping quality of music thus operates on an affective register as music invades or penetrates (*kataduetai*) the depths of one's character. This much is made clear when Aristotle concludes, "therefore it is plain that music has the power of producing a certain effect on the character of the soul" (*Politics* 8.5.10).

Following the line of thinking expounded by Damon, and also by the character Protagoras in Plato's dialogue whereby the rhythms and scales literally "move in" to the soul (*Protagoras* 326B), Aristotle and Plato view music as an almost mystical mode of provoking particular dispositions. In other words, music's capacity to transmit dispositions falls outside the category of reasoned, conscious learning, as rhythms and modes invade the soul and, at times, excite the body to movement. As J. G. Warry describes it, learning from music takes place through the production of tension or relaxation at muscular and nervous levels and is thereby more direct, more powerful than learning through other means (1962: 109). It is precisely because of music's direct, bodily delivery, its capacity for dispositional transformation, according to Aristotle, that he recommends music be used for education, and used prudently. Damon, Aristotle, and Plato therefore all mark music as an *ēthos* delivery system, an affective phusiopoietic mechanism.

The affective quality of the *aulos* makes Aristotle nervous, however, as evidenced by his jittery claim that the *aulos* has an "exciting influence (*orgiastikon*)" (1341a22) and his insistence that the youths of Athens should thus not be taught to play it. (Perhaps this logic explains why the *aulos*-players in gymnasia and palaestra were slaves or attendants.) When describing the effects of the *aulos,* Aristotle uses the word *orgiastikon,* which is another disposition, one with mystical, ecstatic associations, as *orgia* is the noun used to demarcate religious practices and is often associated with Dionysus (*LSJ* 1246).

Still, given Aristotle's trepidations (also supported by Plato's Socrates in the *Republic*), why, then, are *aulos*-players so common as to be almost fixtures in educational spaces? The answer inheres in the very sources of Aristotle's fear. First, because the *aulos* is the facilitator of shuddering, almost violent excitement and emotion (*orgiastika kai pathētika*) (1342b4), it likely provided a kind of incitement to excited movement, a spurring-on of sorts. Moreover, the *aulos*'s mystical quality produces a kind of open malleability of the body and therefore soul, which allows for the easy invasion of rhythms, as suggested by the widespread assumptions about the way music produces *ēthos*. At stake once again in this phusiopoietic mechanism is transformation on a nonconscious level.

Insofar as it performs the time-keeping function for repetition of movements while injecting the soul with forms of character, music combines regulation with seduction as the invasive quality of sound incites the body-mind complex to transform. Since ancient texts have a good deal to say about music in education, and, moreover, what they do say connects explicitly with athletic and rhetorical training methods and dynamics, music provides a useful way to consider rhetorical training as a part of a network of practices. Specifically, as a molder of *ēthos,* music served as a phusiopoietic tool for the ancients and was hence a facilitator of athletic and rhetorical training, insofar as it helped the physical trainers, as Isocrates describes it, set the students at exercises (*Antidosis* 184). As such, attention to music's role in ancient education brings to light the mimetic and repetitive aspects of phusiopoietic training, aspects that emphasize education as a bodily practice and also bring to the fore questions about gendered subject production.

The Three Rs

Music, moreover, calls attention to the "three Rs" of ancient pedagogy: rhythm, repetition, and response. It is these modes of learning, I will suggest, that comprise the sophistic method of rhetorical training. The three Rs thus loop training back to *kairos* and *mētis,* thereby securing the body's critical role in learning and performing.

The Greek word *rhythmos* may be used to indicate "any regular recurring motion" or "measured motion or time." The motion-time complex of meanings then folds into disposition, as *rhythmos* may also mean "symmetry," "state or condition, temper, disposition," "form, shape of a thing," "manner" (*LSJ* 1576). In the range of meanings alone we can see the way in which regulated repetition produces disposition. For Plato, rhythm was tightly bound with order (*taxis*), as he claims that the realm of the bodily order of motion (*kinēseōs taxei*) is known as *rhythmos*. The jump to training is not too far, as we see in Plato's *Phaedrus,* when the character Socrates deploys a noun form of the verb *rhythmizō* (*rhythmizontes*) to indicate education (*Phaedrus* 253B). But it is the kind of education suggested by this peculiar use of the rhythmic verb that matters. In short, rhythm is movement (Anderson 1966: 11), and the direction and manner of movement make all the difference in the context of learning.

As Warry explains, rhythm is derived from the verb meaning "to flow," and the term itself invokes the movement of rivers: "when Greek poets refer to the 'flow' of these seas, they are thinking not only of undulation but of current, and the Greek idea of rhythm is one of current combined with alternation, of continuity with vicissitude" (1962: 115). Here, Warry locates in the ancient concept of rhythm a quality of cyclical differentiation, the same kind of movement Heraclitus invokes in his still-famous saying, "It is not possible to step twice into the same river" (DK 22 B91), for the substances simultaneously combine and scatter (*sunistatai kai apoleipei*). It is the interrelation between the generalized path of the riverbed with its interruptive rocks and sediment, on the one hand, and the force of the water's current, on the other, that produces the eddies and swirls, the sudden shifts in direction within the general flow—herein lies the rhythm. Rhythm therefore produces distinctive movements within a generalized direction; it combines fixity with variability. Put simply, rhythm emerges from difference.[5]

Yet, how do a river's movement and a Heraclitean notion of differentiation help elucidate ancient educational methods? Consider the remnants of the ancient wrestling treatise mentioned in chapter 3. Even though the treatise is from the second century CE, it constitutes a culmination of training methods (Harris 1966: 173) and is the only remaining manual of its kind. The fragment's style—its movement—is quite telling, so I translate it here:

> Set up in the middle and engage the head from the right.
> You envelop him. You get under his hold; You step through,
>   engage (*plexon*).
> You throw him with your right hand.
> You are thrown; having attached from the side you throw left.
> You throw him off with your left hand.
> You turn him around. You entwine. You turn around.
> You engage with a grip on both sides. (Jüthner 1969: 26)[6]

This wrestling treatise illustrates the three Rs of sophistic pedagogy: rhythm, repetition, and response. Even the passage itself takes on an almost hypnotic cadence through the repetition of pointed commands: "You turn him around. You engage (*plexon*)," etc. The logic of the passage seems quite straightforward: by going through micro-motions over and over, the wrestler will acquire a bodily rhythm that enables a forgetting of directives. In other words, as rhythm is achieved, knowledge of fundamentals becomes bodily rather than conscious, and habituation ensues.

This style of teaching emphasizes response as well, as the exercises are performed with an opponent, the "him" of the passage. "You get under his hold; You step through, engage . . . You throw him off with your left hand." Instructed in pairs together (Gardiner 1910: 374), wrestlers in training went through their motions, executing the drill-techniques described in the papyrus fragment above, and as shown on the often-illustrated statue base once built into the wall of Themistocles in Athens (fig. 6.6). This image of paired wrestlers, commonly appear-

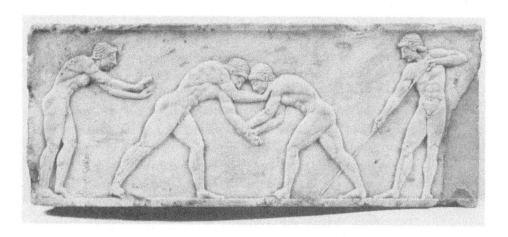

FIGURE 6.6
Scene of wrestlers practicing, from a marble statue base found built
into the wall of Themistocles in Athens: Athens NM 3476.
© National Archaeological Museum, Athens.

ing in vase paintings, shows two wrestlers (center) going through their
motions and as such helps us to visualize the drill-techniques described
above.

Both the statue base and the passage show how responsiveness becomes incorporated in rhythm, as the opponent's moves must be taken
into account, reacted to, and countered, all in the blink of an eye. The
fragment's command *plexon* is noteworthy here, as it can mean "enter-
twine," "engage," or, as Poliakoff suggests, "fight it out" (1987: 52–53).
Hence, the opponent's moves and the attention to specificity they require introduce variation in the repetition, demanding a new move in
between each throwing directive. Stylistically, the manual captures the
difference between repetitions, demanding and producing its own kind
of rhythmic response.

A consideration of rhythm, repetition, and response reintroduces a
consideration of time, as a "nowness" pervades repetition and the difference it produces. Recall from chapter 3 the way in which Philostratus
and Isocrates reiterate the importance of using situational encounters
to teach *kairos*. The repetition of movements is always produced in relation—to the opponent, to one's shadow, to the javelin, to the rhythmic
sounds of the *aulos*—hence the centrality of *kairos,* the time of response,
of singularity, to sophistic pedagogy.

Diligence in Repetition

The three Rs of athletic training—rhythm, repetition, response—lie at the very heart of Isocrates' conception of training. In conjunction with the three Rs style of training, it is worth considering the intensity denoted by the word Isocrates uses for both athletic and rhetorical training—*epimeleias*. The word itself encapsulates several dimensions of *phusiopoiesis* discussed in chapter 4, for it suggests an intense engagement, "diligent attention," "care," and even, in plural form, "pains" (*LSJ* 645). Its root, *meletē,* means "practice," "exercise," and, when used in terms of rhetorical training, often means "declamation" (*LSJ* 1097).

Repetition, rhythm, and diligence were brought together early on in an intense manner by the rhapsodes, who, with their remarkable preservation through memory of Homeric songs and their concomitant role in the transition from oral to written texts (as detailed by Richard Enos), laid the groundwork for rhetoric's emergence as a discipline (Enos 1993: 9–23; see also North 1966: 1–31). Noteworthy too is the amount of diligence that must have been required to become a respected professional rhapsode. With the long hours and effort spent memorizing and repeating poetry, rhapsodes may have been the first to exhibit such intense *epimeleias* and thus should be remembered alongside athletes, next to whom they competed at festivals, as an important model for the kind of rhetorical training that would ultimately be espoused by the sophists and Isocrates.

Aristotle, too, refers to *epimeleias* in a further elaboration of the nature-as-habit doctrine and its relationship to pleasure and pain in the context of educational practices: "Diligent attention (*epimeleias*) and studies (*spoudas*) and exertions (*suntonias*) are painful; for these too are necessarily compulsions unless they become habitual; then habit makes them pleasurable (*ethos poiei hēdu*)" (*Rhetoric* 1370a4; translation adapted from Kennedy 1980). The three nouns here—*epimeleias, spoudas,* and *suntonias*—are almost synonymous in their forces of intensity. *Epimeleias,* as noted above, suggests an intense engagement with or even a "pursuit" of an object so as to take charge of it. The word also has forces of "curator" and "commissioner" (*LSJ* 1645) which link such diligent care to ownership. In this regard, recall the Lyceum inscription examined in the last chapter, bearing the description of Dionysios, "son of Dionysodoros of the Kekropid tribe, overseer (*epimelētēs*) of the

Lyceum" (Travlos 1980: 347). The gymnasiarch's job description entailed diligent vigilance as well.

Spoudas, the second key term in Aristotle's descriptive passage, comes from the word for speed (*spoudē*), and suggests an intensity of pace, a zealous exertion, or earnestness in one's studies. In some cases, it is used to mean "disputation," and thus has affiliations with rhetoric's *agōn.* Similarly, *suntonias* suggests a kind of impetuous vehemence, and offers a way of describing intensity through musical language, where it means "high pitched" or "acute" (*LSJ* 1728).

The learning dynamic described by Aristotle approximates an Empedoclean fragment wherein Empedocles exhorts Pausanias to approach his teachings with a certain intensity:

> If you push them (*ereisas*) firmly under your crowded thoughts (*prapidessin*), and contemplate (*meletēisin*) them favorably with unsullied and constant attention, assuredly all these will be with you through life, and you will gain much else from them, for of themselves they will cause each thing to grow into the character (*auta gar auxei taut' eis ēthos hekaston*), according to the nature (*phusis*) of each. (DK 31 B110; trans. Wright [1981: 258])

This passage is rich with commentary on how education works to sculpt character. Here, Empedocles encourages Pausanias to engage his teachings with a particular intensity, as indicated by the verb *ereisas,* which has the force of push, thrust, and, once again, struggle. Further, Empedocles leaves no room for speculation about the struggle's location—it occurs "under your crowded thoughts (*prapidessin*)." *Prapidessin* marks a spot just under the diaphragm, in the midriff area. According to Liddell and Scott, this area was deemed the somatic seat of intellect, the "mental powers and affections" that helped induce understanding.

Once again, the body plays an important role in Greek thought on habit production. Just as in the instance of musical rhythms, bodily habits emerge from an opening up of the body for such phusiopoietic shaping. It's important to remember, too, that for Empedocles, *mētis,* or cunning intelligence, emerges from the encounter with the immediate (fr. 106; see chapter 2), and the encounter is more than perception—mind meets (and masters) matter—instead, it is a bodily production, a mutually constitutive struggle among bodies and surrounding forces.

As Aristotle's and Empedocles' passages suggest, the struggle habit formation entails is intensely demanding—even violent (as suggested by *bia*, "force," "act of violence")—for it requires sustained engagement, or, as Janet Atwill puts it in her consideration of the same passage, such engagement demands a "severe discipline of contemplation" (1998: 90). In short, this level of engagement requires intensive attention and disciplined, painful, repeated exercise, all forces of *meletē*.

As such, *meletē* becomes the means through which permanent dispositions develop; it is the most effective mode of *phusiopoiesis*. When he discusses the disposition (*hexis*) of self-restraint in *Nicomachean Ethics*, Aristotle considers the relationship between habit, nature, and *meletē*:

> Those who have become unrestrained through habit are more easily cured than those who are unrestrained by nature, since habit is easier to change than nature; for even habit is hard to change, precisely because it is a sort of nature, as Evenus says: "I say practice (*meletēn*) is long-lasting, friend, and moreover with humankind it finally becomes their nature." (7.10.4–5)

As Jeffrey Walker points out in his discussion of the above passage, "*meletē* . . . is a means of cultivating *ēthos*" (2000a: 148). And it is the *kind* of *ēthos* suggested here that makes all the difference. This passage is noteworthy because it suggests that practice produces the very habit of self-control necessary to make oneself capable of training. In other words, the components of *phusiopoiesis*—the readiness, the submission, the painful subjection—are enabled through one's habit of *meletē*, of a resolute belief in the transformative work of practice.

Training, or *epimeleias*, thus occurs through repeated, sustained engagement—a shared trait of athletic and rhetorical training as elaborated by Isocrates in *Antidosis*, where this study began. Recall that for Isocrates, athletic and rhetorical training are "parallel and complementary" (*Antidosis* 182), the means by which "masters prepare the mind to become more intelligent and the body more serviceable" (182). In other words, these twin arts are, for Isocrates, the two most fundamental arts for citizen training, because this particular training juncture enables teachers to "advance their pupils to a point where they are better men and where they are stronger in their thinking or in the use of their bodies" (185).

This mode of teaching thus, in Isocrates' logic, better equips students to become effective citizens. Effective teachers, therefore, do not separate the two kinds of education, but rather use "similar methods of instruction, exercise, and other forms of discipline" (182).

> For when they take on pupils, the physical trainers instruct their followers in the postures (*ta schēmata*) that have been invented for bodily contests, while those whose concern is philosophy pass on to their pupils all the structures that discourse employs. When they have made them experienced with these, and they have discussed them with precision (*diakribōsantes*), they again exercise the students and habituate them to hard work, and then compel them to combine (*suneirein*) everything they have learned. (*Antidosis* 183–85)

Stylistically, this passage performs precisely Isocrates' point about the interrelatedness of the two kinds of training. The first sentence contains two related yet distinct accounts of physical and philosophical training. In the second sentence, however, the two kinds of training merge in style as rhetorical training assumes the very dynamic found in the illustrative wrestling treatise above. The verb *diakribōsantes,* for example, invokes a sense of precision, even perfection, obtained through a minute attention to detail, in this case the minutiae of discursive, bodily movements. Such attention no doubt is enabled through rhythmic repetition of *schēmata,* a term that may be used to describe a wrestling move, a figure of speech, a particular style or manner, or even gesticulation, as in rhetorical delivery (*LSJ* 1745), an important area of inquiry that I will revisit shortly.

But the passage above also connects rhythmic repetition to response production, as Isocrates calls for students to "combine" (*su-neirein*) in practice the *schēmata* "in order that they may grasp them more firmly (*bebaioteron kataschōsi*) and bring their notions (*doxais*) in closer touch with the occasions (*tōn kairōn*) for applying them" (*Antidosis* 184). In other words, at stake in the connection between rhetorical and athletic training for Isocrates is the link between *schēmata*—forms of movement acquired through repetitive habituation—and their use in response to particular situations. Once again, *kairos* comes to the fore as a critical concept taught only through inhabiting situations.

In his *Outline of a Theory for Practice* (1977), Pierre Bourdieu notes that the sophists, when called upon to systematize their arts, came up against "the right way and the right moment—*kairos*—to apply the rules, or as the phrase so aptly goes, to *put into practice* a repertoire of devices or techniques" (20). "To put into practice" aptly describes the aim of Isocrates' pedagogy, and *kairos* is thus one of his primary concerns. As Isocrates contends, no system of knowledge can teach kairotic response; rather such response emerges out of repeated encounters with difference—different opponents in different positions at different times and places.

From *Sunousia* to *Mimēsis:* Becoming by Association

Musical rhythm comes to inhabit the body through productive repetition, as we have seen, and rhythm also operates through a kind of *mimēsis,* another element critical to sophistic pedagogy and another way of producing repeated encounters with difference. As demonstrated earlier, for Aristotle music is doubly mimetic: its rhythms imitate *ēthos,* and when it invades the body and grips the soul, the connection formed between music and listener produces a second *mimēsis,* as the listener imitates ethical rhythms.

Mimēsis, or imitation, was, for most Greeks, a primary mode of learning, as illustrated by Democritus' fragment on acquiring technical expertise through the observation of animals: "We are students of the animals in the most important things: the spider for spinning and mending, the swallow for building, and the songsters, swan and nightingale, for singing, by way of imitation (*kata mimēsin*)" (DK 68 B154). In other words, mimetic learning happens through a relation with someone or something else, an observation and repetition of another's actions and practices.

That imitation was considered a basic part of the pedagogical process in ancient Athens has been well established (Beck 1964: 268; Too 2000: 44–45), and a pithy saying by Democritus puts imitative logic in its most precise form: "One must either be good or imitate a good man" (DK 68 B39). From early on, then, Greek philosophers and poets held that learning happens through alliances. In other words, the forces (people, music, movements) one is subject to will necessarily shape and reshape body and soul. Take, for example, the following lines from Theognis:

> It is good to be called to a feast and sit beside a good man who knows all learning—to associate with him (*tou suniein*) whenever he says

something good so that you might learn and go home holding an advantage (*kerdos*). (*Theognidea* 563–66)

Here, *suniein,* a verb meaning "to come together," "to observe," or "to associate with," is the verbal form of the noun *sunousia,* literally "being together," "habitual or constant association," even "sexual intercourse" (*LSJ* 1723). *Sunousia* produces relations, alliances, which in turn occasion *mimēsis.*

Another Theognidean fragment helps elaborate the nature of such close association, as he advises his friend and protégé Kyrnos:[7]

> Turn (*estrephe*) to all friends, Kyrnos, a variable habit (*poikilon ēthos*), mingling your disposition (*orgēn*) in the manner of each one: now pursue (*ephu*) one, now move toward (*ephepeu*) a disposition of another kind; for skill (*sophiē*) is even more powerful (*kreisson*) than great virtue (*megalēs aretēs*). (*Theognidea* 1071–74)

At first glance, Theognis' advice for obtaining skill seems quite easy: Kyrnos need only spend time with smart people. But the remarkable number of active, imperative, movement-based verbs (*estrephe, ephu, ephepeu*) suggests that Kyrnos' task is far more complex. Recalling from chapter 2 the meanings of *poikilon ēthos*—the changeable, many-colored disposition—it becomes clear that Theognis is telling his friend, once again, to assume an octopus-*ēthos,* to make himself malleable, to open himself up and move toward skillful dispositions he sees in others. Such active movement enables the alliances necessary for phusiopoietic *ēthos* production.

In *Areopagiticus,* Isocrates once again returns to the mechanics of training practiced by his "ancestors" (43), hearkening back to the forces which produced the Democritean and Theognidean observations discussed above. The very best of students, Isocrates contends, didn't spend time in gambling houses or with flute girls, "but remained deliberately devoted (*epitēdeumasin*) to those pursuits they had been assigned, admiring and emulating (*thaumazontes kai zēlountes*) those who excelled in these" (48). What Isocrates pinpoints here is a pedagogy of association—a cultivation of habits and practices achieved by placing oneself in close relation to those who practice the arts one is pursuing; these arts had been named earlier in the treatise as horsemanship, athletics, hunting, and philosophy (45).

The terms *thaumazontes* and *zēlountes,* yoked together in this passage and translated "admiring" and "emulating," work together to link desire to action, as discussed in chapter 4. That is, the observing and admiring lead to an active emulating, an attempt to become like the object of admiration. But *zēlountes* conveys more than imitation (*mimēsis*), for its root verb (*zēloō*), here translated "to emulate," may also be rendered "to vie with." Its connotations, ranging from jealousy and envy to zealous admiration, all hold a kind of desire—to "strive after, affect, desire emulously" (*LSJ* 755). The Isocratean passage thus suggests a concomitant coveting and agonistic striving after qualities embodied in an expert practitioner of the art at hand: repetition can therefore not easily be extricated from response.

Instances of associative pedagogy frequently come from the sophistic characters in Platonic dialogues. Recall (from chapter 4) the way Archaic literature functions to produce the desire to imitate. In the *Protagoras,* the phrasing produces literature as a place into which a youth is sent, as an army is sent to battle (*anagkazousin*); upon "entering" literature, he encounters the descriptions and encomia of good men from the past, so "that the boy in envy (*zēlōn*) may imitate (*mimētai*) them and yearn to become (*ginesthai*) even as they" (326). Again, envy and desire emerge as a necessary component of imitation. But this imitation is given a place—here the literature, for Isocrates, the teacher's instructive milieu—locations the students are to inhabit to the extent that the practices therein begin to inhabit them, as we see in the case of music when the rhythms and scales quite literally move in (*oikeiousthai*) to the boys' souls (326b). Here, envy and desire rename the active, impelling forces operating in Theognis' urgings of Kyrnos.

Isocrates articulates precisely how associative pedagogy fits in with other modes of learning. He writes in *Against the Sophists* that in addition to making the principles of oratory available for students, the teacher should "in himself provide such an example of oratory that the students who have taken shape (*ektupōthentas*) under his instruction and are able to imitate (*mimēsasthai dunamenous*) him will, at once, show in their speaking an unsurpassed degree of grace and charm" (18).

Here the word translated "taken shape," *ektupōthentas,* comes from *ektupos,* a term used in reference to the art of sculpting and meaning "worked in relief" or "formed on a model." The word itself marks the kind of imitation suggested by Isocrates' scheme: one which provides a rough form to be followed in the sculpting of the student. The passive form of the verb is suggestive too, insofar as it thwarts a notion of a "sculptor" per se; the shape, rather, emerges under the teacher's instruction, or in a particular milieu—that is, out of a relational, associative dynamic. In other words, as chapter 4 suggested, the sculpting here emerges from a pedagogical alliance between the model and the student.

Perhaps more important, however, is the way in which the teacher as exemplar functions to supplement "principles of the art" in Isocrates' educational schemes. Indeed, attention to the precise language preceding the passage on imitation suggests that modeling is not "teaching" at all, but rather something quite different: "The teacher must go through these aspects as precisely as possible, so that nothing teachable is left out, but as for the rest, he must offer himself as a model" (*Against the Sophists* 17; trans. Mirhady and Too [2000]). In other words, once the principles have been exhausted, there is still a remainder, a portion of the art of oratory that cannot be transferred through explicit discussion of composition, arrangement, and style (16).

This remainder, which enables students of philosophy to achieve "the perfect disposition" (*teleiōs hexousin*) hearkens back to *kairos*, the time of action, and also at the same time has to do with *manner*, an almost unarticulable style and grace that can be observed and emulated but not easily rendered into precepts. Here, in addition, *teleiōs* is a descriptor used to suggest near-perfection, and also contains the root of *telos* or ultimate goal. Nonetheless, as suggested early on in regard to Pindar's notion of "questing" for *aretē* (chapter 1), the ability to achieve this degree of perfection depends on the constant repetition of a certain *hexis*, here described as a degree of "grace and charm." In other words, the "end result" of such pedagogy is not a finished product, but a dispositional capacity for iteration.

"A Calisthenics of Manhood"

The development of a capacity for iteration began early in the educational process, with deportment training and exercises for young boys (Freeman 1969: 129).[8] In the Archaic and Early Classical periods, training in deportment took on a bodily manner, with attention to self-presentation, bodily carriage, standing, sitting, and walking.

As Maud W. Gleason notes in her study of later sophists, such a focus on the corporeal elements of deportment was central to the production of masculinity in antiquity. It was here, in these youthful exercises, that what Gleason calls "the cultivation of manliness" found its beginnings. As Gleason puts it, "Deportment matters. It is a shorthand that encodes, and replicates, the complex realities of social structure, in a magnificent economy of voice and gesture" (Gleason 1995: xxiv). Gleason's study of the second century CE's treatment of deportment in rhetorical training might be elucidated historically through a consideration of the Archaic and Classical deportment training which took place in the realm of gymnastics, under the watchful eye of the *paidotribēs*. In this light, Gleason's catchy observation, "rhetoric was a calisthenics of manhood" (xxii) takes on a more literal force.

Indeed, bodily comportment was an abiding concern for ancient educators. Aristophanes' *Clouds* provides some insight into the fastidious attention paid to such practices under the "old education," as the character *Kreitton* articulates the relationship between behaving oneself and managing one's body: "Then in the gymnasium, when they sat down, they were expected to keep their legs well up" (line 966). This passage suggests a double force of manner: the politic, behavioral force, where one learned to repeat polite actions, and the way in which that behavior was linked to particular styles of moving: a manner of walking, speaking, acting, standing, and, in the Aristophanic instance, sitting.

This early emphasis on manner and movement carries through all phases of rhetorical and athletic training, as evidenced in the Isocratean passage above where he invokes the perfect disposition in regards to rhetoric, and also in Aeschines' observation (mentioned in this book's introduction) that he and his contemporaries "can recognize an athlete by his bodily vigor (*euexia*) without visiting the gymnasium" (*Against Timarchus* 189).

Underpinning Aeschines' ethical argument here is a habituated practice of bodily reading, a practice Aristotle refers to in *Nicomachean Ethics* when, in his discussion of how wittiness indicates a versatile character, he writes, "We judge men's characters, like their bodies, by their movements (*ek tōn kinēsōn*)" (1128a13–15). And later, in his discussion of *hexis*, Aristotle's logic becomes almost tautological, when he argues that strong dispositional qualities cannot be separated from the status of their source: "healthy walking means walking as a healthy man would walk" (1129a17). While the logic sounds tautological, the practice of bodily reading actually depends on habituation—one knows healthy walking when one sees it, precisely because one has seen a healthy person walking many times before.[9]

Again, repetition conditions the habit of mind, this time by shaping the way one person reads another's movements. The *euexia*, literally the "good bodily habits," of the athlete and the "perfect disposition" (*teleiōs hexousin*) of a rhetor both emerged from cultural values and practices—from an inexplicable sense of what constitutes a good athlete or a good rhetor. Noteworthy, however, is the way in which the "sense" is generally tied to singular examples, *paradeigmata,* specific instantiations of good actions. Both the athlete's and the rhetor's *euexia,* as evident in Aristotle's direct comparison, overlapped, informed, and indeed helped produce each other.

As such, athletics and rhetoric were bodily arts concerned with dispositional training, for as Cicero wrote centuries later, "*Est enim actio quasi sermo corporis* (by action the body talks)" (*de Oratore* 3.59.222). Here, rhetorical delivery exhibits quite clearly the convergence of these bodily arts.

Cheironomia

Early training in deportment was inextricable from a kind of bodily training in "gesticulation," to *cheironomein* (Freeman 1969: 129), literally, the custom of hand movement, and also the term for "shadowboxing," a training practice whereby a boxer rehearses and observes his jabs and punches, quite literally by sparring with his shadow (a shadow boxer is pictured in figure 6.3).

Cheironomia became associated with training in rhetorical delivery, as young men learned to combine the force of their gestures with the direction of their speech. Delivery, the aspect of rhetoric that deals with voice, gestures, and other elements of presentation, was the rhetorical "canon" most obviously concerned with corporeality.[10]

As a recent article by Christopher Johnstone (2001) points out, despite its having been considered the most important aspect of rhetoric among the ancients, delivery is a category drastically overlooked in contemporary histories of rhetoric (121–25). Johnstone's work relies on archaeological and textual evidence to argue that delivery was likely a focus of sophistic pedagogy in the fifth century BCE, and he writes compellingly about the sheer bodily strength required to deliver powerful, effective speeches at venues such as the Pnyx, the large outdoor area where citizens gathered to deliberate legal and political matters (129–31). Perhaps one reason for this oversight is delivery's sheer corporeality, as well as its attention to the less rational qualities of rhetorical speeches such as volume, rhythm, and cadence.

Quintilian, writing nearly five centuries after the early sophists, located Roman oratory's indebtedness to gymnastics firmly in the domain of delivery:

> I do not think there is any cause to blame those who have found a little time also for the teachers of gymnastics. But the same name applies to those who train gesture and movement to ensure that the arms are held straight, the hands show no lack of education and no country-bred manners, the stance is proper, there is no clumsiness in moving the feet, and the head and eyes do not move independently of the general inclination of the body. No one will deny that these matters come under Delivery, or attempt to separate Delivery from the person of the orator. Nor, of course, should anyone disdain to learn what he ought to do, especially as "*chironomy*," which, as its name tells us, is *the law of gesture,* originated in heroic times and was approved by the greatest Greeks. (*Institutio Oratorio* 1.11.16–19; trans. Russell)

Here Quintilian articulates a critical intersection between rhetoric and athletics: the art of delivery. Quintilian described appropriate delivery as balanced, poised, emitting elegance, exuding propriety.

These qualities, Aristotle claimed, could be learned from drama; indeed, the Greek word for delivery, *hypokrisis,* also meant acting. But Cicero locates the roots of delivery elsewhere; in *de Oratore,* the character Crassus disagrees with the Aristotelian genealogy when he claims:

> But all these emotions must be accompanied by gesture—not this stagy gesture reproducing the words but one conveying the general situation and idea not by demonstration but by hints, with this vigorous manly (*virili*) throwing out of the chest, borrowed not from the stage and the theatrical profession but from the parade ground or even from wrestling. (*de Oratore* 3.59.220; trans. Sutton and Rackham)

Further, the practice of shadowboxing, or *cheironomia,* invoked by Crassus here, itself combines agonism, imitation, and the three Rs —rhythm, repetition, and response—and as such provided a useful model for rhetorical training. The Athenian stranger of Plato's *Laws* invokes this training technique as an analogue for the training of citizens, whom he refers to as "competitors in the greatest contests (*athlētas tōn megistōn*)":

> If we were boxers, for a great many days before the contest we should have been learning (*emanthanomen*) how to fight, and we would work hard, imitating all we would intend to employ when fighting for victory, thus approximating the real thing as nearly as possible . . . and if we chanced to be very short of training companions, do you suppose that we would be deterred by fear of senseless laughter from hanging up a lifeless dummy and practicing on it? Indeed, if ever we were anywhere without either live or lifeless training companions, would we not undergo shadow-fighting (*skia-machein*) against ourselves? How else do you suppose shadowboxing (*cheironomein*) would have come into being? (8.830b–c)

As in many instances of citizen-training considered so far in this study, this passage suggests that only the *agōn* can prepare one fully for the *agōn*, as evidenced by the question posed before this passage: "Suppose we had been training boxers or pankratiasts or competitors in any similar branch of athletics, should we have moved into the contest without previously engaging in daily combat with someone?" (830a–b). Here, regular combat provides the repetition necessary for learning, and *cheironomia* exemplifies the role of agonism in training: even the self can be the other in agonistic preparation.

Furthermore, the passage suggests the way in which *cheironomein*, in addition to being a practice of productive repetition, is also a mode of imitation by which one approximates the agonistic situation, rehearsing previously observed bodily moves and gestures in an imagined context. For Plato's Athenian stranger, the athlete provides a useful model for citizens-in-training insofar as he makes use of any available means of agonistic engagement.

The Case of Demosthenes

As Cicero and Quintilian suggest, however, the connection between athletics and rhetoric goes much deeper, as training in public presentation was firmly rooted in gymnastic training. It is here, in the practice of rhetorical delivery, that the bodily arts of athletic and rhetorical training fused most noticeably. And it is also in this fusion where the implications for gender and identity formation become most apparent.

At stake in delivery's connection to athletics, as Cicero's text makes clear, is a certain conception of "manliness," indicated by a particular kind of carriage, a vigorous manner, recognizable by sight and solidly associated with the deportment of athletes, the *euexia* invoked by Aeschines. Let us turn briefly to the example of Demosthenes' rhetorical training, invoked by many figures of late antiquity as a telling model of dedicated, agonistic learning.

According to most sources, Demosthenes overcame numerous shortcomings, not the least of which was his puny body, attributed to his mother's insistence that he not work so hard in the palaestra (Diogenes Laertius 3.4). As a boy, he was dubbed "Batalus," a nickname with a couple of associations. First, as Aeschines avers in a common ad hominem move, the nickname marks his "effeminacy and lewdness" (*Against Timarchus* 131); Diogenes Laertius supports this contention by observing that Batalus was the name of an effeminate *aulos*-player. The second association refers to Demosthenes' speech impediment, for *Batalos* also means "stammerer" in Greek. Demosthenes was widely known to have a pronounced stutter, so pronounced, Cicero's Antonius contends, that he could not even pronounce the letter R of the art he claimed to practice (*de Oratore* 1.61.260).

Nonetheless, as the stories go, Demosthenes convinced his tutor to allow him to observe the famous Callistratus in the law courts, at which point "Demosthenes conceived a desire to emulate his fame," and "bidding farewell to his other studies and to the usual pursuits of boyhood, he practiced himself laboriously in declamation, with the idea that he too was to be an orator" (Diogenes Laertius 5.3–5). Here, in his description of Demosthenes' training, Diogenes Laertius relates a story of *phusiopoiesis* and its components—of the seduction, commitment, and diligent practice such transformation of one's nature requires.

As Plutarch tells it, such seduction was accompanied by a sense of shame, as his early rhetorical endeavors were ridiculed by crowds as well as by respected citizens. Describing the events following one particularly distressing incident, Plutarch writes:

When he had left the assembly and was wandering about dejectedly in the Piraeus, Eunomus the Thrasian, who was already a very old man, saw him and scolded him because, although he had a style of speaking which was like that of Pericles, he was throwing himself away out of weakness and lack of courage, neither facing the multitude with boldness, nor preparing his body for these forensic contests, but suffering it to wither away in slothful neglect. (*Life of Demosthenes* 848.4)[11]

At stake in Eunomus' critique of Demosthenes is a notion of masculine self-care, a sense of the good kind of body (*euexia*) a strong, manly speaker should cultivate in order to be prepared for the contests, the *agōnas* of the law courts.

Plutarch also describes another moment as formative for Demosthenes, when Demosthenes, once again dejected about his performance, lamented to Satyrus that while he had "used up the vigor of his body" on this particular occasion, he still was unable to "hold the bema," or maintain the assembly floor. Satyrus then offers to explain to Demosthenes why this is so, but his offer takes the form of agonistic demonstration, as Satyrus challenges Demosthenes to "recite off-hand . . . some narrative speech from Euripides or Sophocles." When Demosthenes complies, Satyrus follows with his own version of the same speech, "reciting it with such appropriate sentiment and disposition that it appeared to Demosthenes to be quite another" (849.2). Convinced, as Plutarch tells it, of the importance of the "delivery and disposition of his words," Demosthenes built what Plutarch calls a "subterranean study" (*oikodomēsai meletētērion*), which became his locus for self-discipline, his site for phusiopoietic transformation.

A central part of Demosthenes' phusiopoietic quest was therefore keen attention to elements of bodily delivery, as he is reputed to have treated his stutter by making it "his habit to slip pebbles into his mouth, and then declaim a number of verses at the top of his voice and without drawing a breath, and this not only as he stood still, but while walking about, or going up a steep slope" (Cicero, *de Oratore* 1.61.261; trans. Sutton and Rackham). Diogenes Laertius also relates the pebble story and adds that Demosthenes exercised his voice by running uphill and reciting speeches in a single breath (11.1–2). "Moreover," adds Diogenes, "he had in his house a large mirror, and in front of this he used to stand and go through his exercises in declamation" (11.2).

This kind of bodily training for rhetorical performance certainly requires *meletē,* a fastidious attention to the art in practice, a shadowboxing of sorts. When Demosthenes practiced in front of the mirror, for example, such practice forced an encounter with the observant other—in this case himself. Self-observed, diligent rehearsal, through repetition, refines the rhythm and develops one's capacity to respond in a particular manner—in this case without a stutter, and in a confident, "manly" way. Such practice, then, operates much like the practice of shadowboxing described by the Athenian stranger in Plato's *Laws.*

Not only was Demosthenes' mode of training corporeal, but in his quest to achieve the bodily vigor and manner of presentation exhibited by Satyrus and others, he enforced his own study in his *meletētērion,* to which, according to Plutarch,

> he would descend every day without exception in order to form his action and cultivate his voice, and he would often remain there even for two or three months together, shaving one side of his head in order that shame might keep him from going abroad even though he greatly wished to do so. (*Life of Demosthenes* 849.1)

Apparent in this compelling description are several elements of *phusiopoiesis.* Demosthenes, made ready through encounters with his failure to perform, as well as his seductive encounters with the likes of Satyrus and Callistratus, subjected himself to difficult training practices, even disfiguring his appearance by shaving one side of his head, in order to ensure the committed *meletē* necessary to transform his nature, to make "Batalus," the styleless weakling, into what Plato's Eleatic stranger might call "an athlete in the contest of words" (*Sophist* 231e).

Demosthenes' training thus emerged out of agonism with others—including himself as other—through which he produced what we might call the meletic spirit, the convergence of desire for transformation, the commitment to practice, and the forcing of regular encounters with the other. Indeed, when describing Demosthenes' rhetorical training, Plutarch compares him to an athlete in training:

> And just as Laomedon the Orchomenian—so we are told—practiced long-distance running by the advice of his physicians, to ward off some disease of the spleen, and then, after restoring his health in this way, entered the great games and became one of the best runners of the long course, so Demosthenes . . . by this means of

acquired ability and power in speaking . . . [and] as it were in the great games, won first place among the citizens who strove with one another (*agōnizomenōn*) on the bema. (*Life of Demosthenes* 848.3)

The stories Plutarch and Diogenes Laertius tell about Demosthenes present him as the "self-made man," the one who overcame "natural" impediments by transforming his countenance and reshaping his disposition. While Demosthenes' is often read as a story of individual merit, the dynamics in his training practices, with their strong connections to the body and roots in gymnastic training, suggest that Demosthenes' "self-fashioning" cannot be considered separately from the forces which produced it: the rejection at the hands of crowds around the bema, the seeking out of models in Callistratus and Satyrus, even — and especially — the "retreat" into the *meletētērion*. Demosthenes' *meletētērion*, therefore, did not function as a cocoonlike private interior space of transformation, but rather as a space for gathering of productive, transformative forces, a phusiopoietic ecology.

While delivery provides an obvious site where rhetoric and athletics converge, it is not the only place where athletic and rhetorical training and their shared status as bodily arts apply. Indeed, as this study suggests, all aspects of sophistic training were bodily to some degree, particularly with their emphasis on rhythm, repetition, and response-production, which together comprise the guiding theory of habituation central to *phusiopoiesis*. Perhaps this is why Demosthenes considered delivery to occupy the first, second, and third most important elements of rhetorical training.

This consideration of Demosthenes suggests that underpinning the phusiopoietic economy is a whole relation to the self that always depends on networks of others. As an example, the conceptions of "manly" delivery that inhere in various critiques of Demosthenes' early rhetorical performances are tightly linked to a kind of bodily reading practice elaborated by Aristotle in his version of the healthy man walking, and to the kind of "questing" after *aretē* elaborated by Pindar, discussed in chapter 1.

In other words, repetition inhabits rhetorical training from several directions. First, the desirable qualities — deportment, carriage, bodily movement — are repeated by others and after constant association with these manners. Through association one acquires a habit of "body-reading," of perceiving desirable qualities and their concomitant values.

If, as Cicero says, the body talks through action—a habituated action—then "body-reading," or the encounter with these actions, emerges as an important (and necessary) effect of such repetition. Such repetition, always in relation to the particular temporal and spatial situation, is therefore productive, insofar as it shapes reading practices and the imitative, repetitive practices that emerge as reading hooks into desire for *sunousia,* for transformation by association.

All styles of repetition, because they are particular to time, space, and the singular cluster of forces enacting them, emerge in response to specific forces: to opponents, to values, beliefs, and practices that shape and are shaped by the differential, emergent repetition. In short, repetition in sophistic-style rhetorical training is always bound up with responsiveness within particular contexts.

Demosthenes' regular, repetitive descent into the *meletētērion* provides an example of a multiply layered response: in this way, his diligence can be read as a response to previous responses to his "lame" presentation style; the response is also impelled by desire to emulate the likes of Callistratus, connected to circulating notions of honor and shame, and the cultural imperative to present a remarkably masculine set of practices: strength of body, prominence, and fluid rhythm of voice, qualities associated with courage, manliness, good disposition, the *euexia* of the athlete—in short, with strong, muscular citizenship.

Rhetorical performance and its concomitant training practices both took place at the level of the body. At stake in bodily performance is an attention to manner—to the *way* in which one acquires artistic expertise—over matter, here meaning subject matter, as in the modern notion of three Rs. That is, rather than focusing on material learned—the sophists didn't have a curriculum in the modern sense of a "subject matter" to be "covered"—sophistic pedagogy emphasized the materiality of learning, the corporeal acquisition of rhetorical movements through rhythm, repetition, and response. This manner of learning-doing entails "getting a feel for" the work—following and producing a rhythm. The body itself becomes a *sundromos,* an intensive gathering of forces (of desire, of vigorous practice, of musical sounds, of corporeal codes), trafficked through and by neurons, muscles, and organs. Entwined with the body in this way, rhetorical training thus exceeds the transmission of "ideas," and rhetoric the bounds of "words."

The next chapter will expand this consideration of bodily habits and body-reading into a look at the cultural habits and practices of athletics and rhetoric in the celebratory festivals and funerals of the Greeks. Such a move will circle back to the *agōn* while opening up an interrogation of the public (read: visible, readable, honorable) Greek body.

The Visible Spoken

Rhetoric, Athletics, and the Circulation of Honor

> Oh, those Greeks! They knew how to live. What is required for that
> is to stop courageously at the surface, the fold, the skin, to adore
> appearance, to believe in forms, tones, words, in the whole Olympus
> of appearance. Those Greeks were superficial—*out of profundity.*
> —Nietzsche, *The Gay Science* (1974a: 38)

In many ways, the instances of bodily reading and production considered in the last chapter—Aeschines' remark about the athlete's recognizable body, Aristotle's comment about knowing a healthy man's walk by virtue of having seen it repeatedly, and the oft-repeated story of Demosthenes' development as an orator through observation—turn on a logic of the visible. The visible, in turn, depends on the knowable, an associative knowledge of bodies: Aristotle's perceiver, for example, must recall instances of healthy men walking, and such recalling requires a prior articulation of walking style as healthy. Aeschines' example invokes the cultural knowledge of what an athletic body looks like, and Demosthenes sees, observes, and tries to emulate orators.

While Aristotle's healthy man walking is a rather mundane example, a similar logic of visibility nonetheless drives the more remarkable, spectacular aspect of Greek culture—that of the festival. This chapter will be set against the backdrop of the Athenian festival, as the festival provided an important cultural context for linking athletics and rhetoric as bodily arts of honor production.

Simply pointing out this cultural-historical link, however, doesn't seem quite sufficient. As bodily arts, rhetoric and athletics are differently infused with the elements of what Nietzsche characterizes as "a whole Olympus of appearances." Decipherable in Nietzsche's bold (if nostalgic) description is a spectacular logic, an economy of appearances that depends on apparent bodily manifestations of the kind of training this book has thus far delineated. Noteworthy, though, is Nietzsche's description of appearance's superficiality as a belief in "forms, tones, words": that which is seen, heard, and said. The economy of appearance is most strikingly present in ancient festivals and competitions, for it is these events that, for the Greeks, most explicitly foregrounded honor and glory through the sights, sounds, and words about which Nietzsche writes.

Within the festival context, athletics and rhetoric inhabit distinctive modalities of appearance: athletics resides more in the realm of the visual, while rhetoric, of course, deals with words. But the curious moments are when the two come together; when what is seen enters into a relation with what is said. As distinct modalities of appearance, rhetoric and athletics help sketch out the complicated relations between "forms" and "words"—the visible and the articulable.

In his consideration of vision from antiquity to the present, Martin Jay argues that a Greek privilege of vision was not only responsible for the subordination of touch, smell, taste, and hearing, but that it also meant—indeed, was premised upon—the denigration of language (1993: 33). With this contention, Jay attributes to vision's reign a corresponding disparaging of rhetoric as associated with the sophists. The ancient festival, though, yields a different story: here, the visible becomes partnered to the rhetorical in ways that complicate Jay's claim considerably. As a modality of appearance, the rhetorical has its own distinct register of visibility, and further, through its ability to move, it supplements the axis of sight by reactualizing what was seen. Put simply, seeing and telling were more mutually constitutive for the Greeks than Jay's account would have us believe.

Instead of trumpeting vision's triumph over language, as Jay would have it, ancient festivals featured a mingling of sights, tones, and words. In the festival context, rhetoric became sutured to athletics precisely through the broader relation between the visible and the articulable: that which is known through bodies, and that which is known through words about these bodies. Before returning to the question of the visible in relation to rhetoric, though, I want first to consider the spectacle of the festival itself.

Rhetoric, Athletics, Festivals

Historians of classical rhetoric have on a number of occasions pointed out the importance of festivals as a context for rhetoric's development in antiquity. Richard Leo Enos, for example, discusses festivals and their importance for the rhapsodic tradition, a precursor to rhetorical practices in Enos' scheme (1993: 18). Along these same lines, W. K. C. Guthrie suggests that sophistic activity at festivals provides evidence that the sophists "considered themselves to be in the tradition of the poets and rhapsodes" (1971: 42), a connection elaborated more fully by Jeffrey Walker (2000a).

John Poulakos discusses festivals briefly in an account of rhetoric's relation to spectacles (1995: 39–44), but lingers instead on the spectacle of drama, thus following Aristotle's logic that rhetorical delivery should be considered in the same light as acting (*Rhetoric* 3.1.8). Scott Consigny offers perhaps the most considered account of the festival as a venue for Gorgias' rhetorical performances, giving special attention to both their agonistic and "theatrical" features (2001: 195–97).

The tendency, by and large, is to focus on rhetoric's relation to poetic and dramatic performances in the festival context. This tendency is understandable, since these genres operate in the discursive milieu, and since there are historical and cultural connections between drama and rhetoric (e.g., Aristotle's account of delivery as acting discussed in the last chapter).[1] But how did these discursive practices relate to the athletic games so central to the circulation of honor? As it turns out, in this context, rhetoric had a rather uneasy connection to athletic performance, one that reveals the tangled relation between visibility and articulability.

A love for spectacle persisted most strenuously at Athens. According to Thucydides, Pericles observed that Athens, more than any other city, provided respite from daily activities in the spectacular games and sacrifices at festivals; the profound pleasure derived from the goodness of the outward appearance (*euprepesin*), as Pericles puts it, caused pain to be sent away (*lupēron ekplessei*) (Thuc. 2.38). Isocrates, too, in *Panegyricus,* a speech written and circulated as a pamphlet at the Olympic festival in 380 BCE (Mirhady, Papillon, and Too 2000: 5), elaborated Athens' "zest for the festival" (44), for Athens, in Isocrates' words, "affords the most numerous and the most admirable spectacles (*theamata pleista)*" (*Panegyricus* 45): Athenian festivals were self-purportedly the most frequent, the best, and the biggest.

It is within a spectacular framework of the spectacle that Isocrates locates the movement of *philotimia*, a profound love of honor (here in verb form, *philotimēthōsin*). The orator marvels at the sheer multitude of people who visit Athens for festivals. Such a gathering, he contends, enables "the most faithful friendships" and "the most varied social interaction" (*Panegyricus* 45); also, and perhaps more important, the festival produced a gathering of onlookers to witness "contests not alone of speed and strength, but of eloquence and wisdom and of all the other arts" (46). These gatherings, with all their variegated activities, social connections, participants, and spectators, thus occasioned a furious celebration of and—by extension—circulation of honor. The ancient festival, that is, constituted a space of visibility that showcased honor (*timē*) precisely by facilitating its exchange. Exchange of honor, as Isocrates makes clear, happened through athletic and rhetorical displays. Isocrates therefore articulates a critical connection between athletics and rhetoric: they both occasion gathering and witnessing.

As Isocrates indicates, athletic contests bring to light the aggregative quality of the festival, *athroisthentōn*, which operates on a logic of display (*epideixis*) and beholding (*theōria*). According to Isocrates, everyone present finds in the festival some aspect which produces a love of honor (*philotimēthōsin*): "the spectators when they see the athletes struggling for their benefit, the athletes when they consider that all have come for their beholding" (*Panegyricus* 44). It is thus the act of beholding, *theōrian*, that produces the performance and enables the production of honor, *timē*.

This important section of *Panegyricus* suggests that rhetorical performance emerged within a network of long-standing ritual practices and, perhaps more interesting, that these ritual practices produced a visible rendering of the abstract—in this case, of honor, glory, virtuosity, and respect. This visible rendering makes Athenian culture into what Goldhill calls "a culture of viewing" (1998: 108). Yet to be considered here, though, are the specific ways in which festivals as networks of spectacles shaped rhetoric as an art of performance, one that is immediately bound up with the articulation and circulation of honor (*timē*), virtue (*aretē*), and fame (*kleos*).

The title of Isocrates' *Panegyricus* turns on the different senses of the *panegyr-* root; its verbal form means "to attend a festival," and by Isocrates' time it had also come to mean "to deliver a speech in public." More generally, different forms of the root can mean "a crowd or audience," and even "display." Packed into the very word for festival, then, are the focal points of this chapter: the festival itself and the act of display and its visual logic, the function of the crowd, the practice of ritualized celebration, and the work of rhetoric to draw these elements together. First, though, it is important to consider why festivals served as a fulcrum of civic interaction and how the visual operated as such a crucial modality of appearance.

A Feast for the Eyes: The Festival

Isocrates makes clear the relation between Athens and its celebrations when he writes, "Our city throughout all time is a festival" (*Panegyricus* 46). As translator George Norlin notes, "festival followed upon festival in Athens, and Isocrates' statement is almost literally true" (1982: 146 n. c). In Athens, as much as one-third of the calendar year was set aside for festival activity (Neils 1992b: 13).[2] It is therefore unsurprising that the Athenians, according to the Old Oligarch, celebrated more festivals than the inhabitants of any other Greek state (Old Oligarch, *Constitution of Athens* 3.8).

The frequency and variety of Athenian festivals didn't so much provide a reprieve from daily life (as Neils would suggest) as constitute its own set of almost daily activities. It was the festival calendar in relation to which the political calendar was drawn up: each lunar moon was given the name associated with a particular festal rite, thereby yielding the Athenian calendar.[3] By Aristotle's time, the Panathenaia—the largest Athenian festival—had its own elected officials (*Ath. Con.* 60.1), and all festivals had to an extent become legislative and logistical ordeals.[4] It seems clear that ancient Athenians repeatedly made spectacles of themselves.[5]

Not only were festivals repeated on a yearly basis, but each was quite elaborate. Each festival was associated with a different deity and was characterized by endless variations on sacrificial and feasting practices (Parke 1977: 183). Also, each usually contained some form of a procession (*pompē*) marking the beginning of celebration, a sacrifice, consumption of meat, and contests of the athletic, musical, poetic, and oratorical variety.

The festal procession stands as the temporal and spatial marker of the festival, as Walter Burkert writes, "The fundamental medium of group formation is the procession, *pompē*. The active participants separate themselves from the amorphous crowd, fall into formation, and move towards a goal, though the demonstration, the interaction with the onlookers, is scarcely less important than the goal itself. Hardly a festival is without its *pompē*" (1985: 99). Particularly salient in Burkert's description is the *pompē*'s role in the production of an ordered spectacle. Further, though, Burkert's point renders explicit the critical relational quality of the procession facilitated by the spectacle: as the spatial and temporal markers of the festival, the *pompai* lent order precisely by articulating the spectator/performer dynamic on a logic of display (Goldhill 1999: 21). The word *pompē*, after all, is also imbued not only with the meaning of "procession" but also with a sense of magnificence, triumph, and even ostentation.

Such features of the *pompē* are illustrated by the central focus of the procession during the Panathenaic festival: the delivery and dedication of the robe commemorating Athena's birthday, the very reason for the festive occasion. Aristotle's account suggests that the elected "stewards of the games," in addition to organizing the festival's procession and contests, were to oversee the production of the festival's *peplos,* a colorful woolen robe made and decorated by women of the community to be carried to and placed on Athena's statue on the Acropolis. What started as a human-size tapestry, however, each year was made larger and larger until it reached a colossal size and had to be transported to the Parthenon as the mast of a wheeled ship (Parke 1977: 39; Neils 1992a: xx; Barber 1992: 113–14).[6] The transport of the *peplos* in the procession thus became a way to display the dazzling dedicatory gift in honor of the city's central deity.

Following the *pompē*, the festival events contained elements of display as well. The Panathenaic festival even held a contest in "manly beauty," the *euandria*. While not much is known about the *euandria*, Aristotle does mention that the prize for the victor was a shield—the Greek marker of manliness *par excellence* (*Ath. Con.* 60.3). Athenaeus writes that in the *euandriais,* the contestant thought to be most beautiful, *kallistous,* was selected as a winner (*Deipnosophistai* 13.565f), and Xenophon (*Memorabilia* 3.3.13) indicates that strength and size were valued in the contest. The *euandria,* therefore, was a celebration of manhood through and through (Crowther 1985: 286–87; Kyle 1992: 95).

The very existence of such a competition in the Panathenaia points to the primary function of the festival: to provide an occasion for gathering wherein material and bodily manifestations of honor may be at once displayed and proclaimed honorable. More common than the *euandria,* though, as the *Panegyricus* suggests, were competitive performances of sports, songs, poems, and even speeches.

The colorful array of spectacles in this festival—the massive, sail-like *peplos* being transported in an equally spectacular procession up to the Acropolis, the exhibition of manliness, and the competitive performers of all stripes—everywhere reinforces the relation between display and proclamation. Plato declares that the value of such gatherings lies precisely in the rendering visible of actions: "for when the habits of men are hidden (*tropois*) from one another in darkness rather than light, no one will gain either his due honor (*timēs*) or office, or the appropriate amount of justice" (*Laws* 738e). According to Plato, the festal gathering provides the "light"—the rendering visible of that which is honorable and good—by providing an occasion for the bodily production of such values.

But light is only part of the story. That is, light (read: visibility) must accompany repeated, recognizable acts, acts known as honorable or good, which is likely why the festival requires such carefully, frequently, and fabulously repeated displays: the valuation is secured through the repetition of festive acts, thus forming a cultural bodily knowledge that binds performers to onlookers.

Celebrations of Death

The bond between performers and onlookers becomes most salient in the instance of funerary celebrations. In ancient Athens, festival and funeral were tightly linked cultural rituals: in fact, many of the practices found in festivals were derived from private funerary rites, which likely preceded the institutionalization of festivals.[7]

Athletic contests are the best and most certain instance of such crossover;[8] literary evidence suggests that funeral games date back to pre-Homeric times. Indeed, by Homer's time, games had already become a kind of poetic *topos.* As William Hailey Willis' study of contests in epic suggests, Homer's lengthy account of the funeral games for Patroclus in *Iliad* Book 23 very likely followed an almost formulaic presence of game motifs in early rhapsodic poetry.[9] We know too that Hesiod recited his poems at the funeral games for Amphidamas in Chalkis (*Works and Days* 654–59).

Most festivals are thought to have evolved from funerary contests in honor of deities and heroes—the Olympic Games, for example, were associated with funerary contests in honor of Pelops (Roller 1981: 107; Pindar *Ol.* 1.90–96; Dionysius of Halicarnassus 5.1.4). The pre-Archaic cultural/poetic formula is simple: death of a hero calls for funeral games. As Achilles pointedly instructs his troops while they prepare for Patroclus' funerary games, "these are the solemn honors owed the dead" (*Iliad* 23.10). These "solemn honors" triangulated between the performers, the onlookers, and the dead.

Early funeral celebrations, while elaborate, were organized privately and occurred on a smaller scale. In the fifth century, however, on the heels of the Second Persian War (479 BCE), the Athenians instituted public funeral games (*agōna ton epitaphion*) for their war dead. According to Diodorus Siculus, in addition to holding the funeral games for the first time, the citizens of Athens also "passed a law that laudatory addresses (*encomia*) upon men who were buried at the public expense should be delivered by speakers selected for each occasion" (11.33.3).[10] And so it was that rhetorical and athletic performance became yoked together as official modes of bestowing honor upon the war dead.

An oration attributed to Aspasia by Socrates in Plato's *Menexenus* discusses these public funerary rituals under the rubric of "care bestowed by the city (*tēs de poleōs tē epimeleian*)" (248e7–8):

> And the city does not ever fail to pay honor to the dead heroes themselves, since the city itself celebrates publicly every year for all those customs performed for each one (individually); and moreover, it establishes contests in athletics and horse-racing and all music. (*Menexenus* 249b3–6)

The speech under consideration is itself a funeral oration, the kind of which Diodorus Siculus writes, marking the legislated public lamentation for the city's dead. Together with the athletic and musical contests of which Plato's Socrates' Aspasia speaks, the oration performs the aforementioned "care bestowed by the city" by articulating the city and its values repeatedly and regularly, *hekaston eniauton* (249b5).

As Nicole Loraux observes, the funeral oration, or the *epitaphios*, "is a political genre in which, governed by civic laws, the logos becomes in turn a civic norm for speaking of Athens. From epitaphios to epitaphios, a certain idea that the city wishes to have of itself emerges" (1986: 14). Such commentary on the city's care of itself via an iterative production of its reputation may also be found in Lysias' funeral oration. In this case, the care of the city becomes manifest in the praise and care of its war dead, those who, as Lysias puts it, risked their lives for "the greatest and noblest ends" (*Funeral Oration* 79.7–80.1). He continues:

> For I say their memory can never decay, their honor enviable by all. By nature they are mourned as mortal, through *aretē* they are praised as immortal. Thus you give them a public funeral, and contests of strength and knowledge and wealth held for them; because we think that those who have fallen in war are worthy of receiving the same honors as immortals. (*Funeral Oration* 79.6–80.5)

Beyond implicitly praising Athens for its capacity to bestow honor, this passage also delineates the logic of funerary contests—and contests in general, for that matter. It is clear, for example, that *agōnes* were a means of keeping *timē* in circulation, whether for the recently dead or for the festival's deity. For the Athenians, the way to give honor and to commit honor to memory was to continually produce it, so they commemorated an honorable death by generating a different kind of *timē* among themselves in the absence of honor once visible.

This tendency to produce a different kind of honor in the absence of the once-visible operates in *epitaphioi* as well: at the completion of Socrates' account of Aspasia's oration, for example, Menexenus responds with overwhelming praise, not of the war dead in the speech, but rather of Aspasia's apparent ability to produce such a fine speech (*Menexenus* 249d). Menexenus' response suggests that those listening to funeral orations listened not merely to hear reasons for bemoaning the dead, but also—and perhaps more important—to decide whether the speech is itself honorable. Hence, at the opening of his *Funeral Oration,* Lysias observes, "while my speech is about these men, my contest is not with their deeds, but with the speakers who have preceded me in praising them" (2.6).

The speeches and contests at funerals were not only iterative—proclaiming honor again and again—but they were also, through their differentiated modes of honor production (athletics, music, rhetoric), novel: they replaced a prior honor with a different kind of honor, thus redirecting honor's circulation from the dead to those who are living, albeit in the name of the dead. The differentiated honors of athletic games and of speeches thus worked together to actualize the magnitude of *timē* achieved, and to ensure that the possibility of honor had not been evacuated with death. Contests and speeches thus helped honor reappear through a new mode, replacing the loss with an inspired assurance that honor still circulated.

But assuming the obvious—that athletics and rhetoric were not identical practices—how, specifically, did these athletic contests and eulogies work to secure honor differently from each other? The *Epitaphios* of Demosthenes suggests that they operate on distinctive registers. In a self-proclaimed interruptive moment (13.1–2), Demosthenes pauses, "before making visible the deeds of these men" (*pepragmena tois andrasi dēloun*), to explain the workings of speech in comparison with the spectacle of the contest:

> For if I had been appointed to adorn [this burial] by spending money or by arranging some other kind of spectacle (*allēn theōrian*) of equestrian or gymnastic contests, the greater my zeal and the more lavish my spending in preparing such spectacles, the better I should have been thought to have met my duty. Having been chosen, however, to commend these men with speech, unless I take my hearers with me, I fear that because of my eagerness I may do the very opposite of what was fitting. For wealth and speed and strength and all other such things hold sufficient advantage in themselves, and they prevail, even if not one of the others wishes it. On the other hand, persuasion with words is bound to the goodwill of the hearers so that even if the speech be moderate, it brings glory and procures favor, but without this, even to speak most fairly (*legein kalōs*) offends the listeners. (*Epitaphios* 14)

Here Demosthenes comments on the necessity of the listeners' active participation in his (and hence the city's) aim to honor the dead, even intimating that if the listeners do not already participate in the economy of honor at hand, then his speech is doomed to failure from the outset. Demosthenes, by claiming that a successful speech is a collective effort, thus attempts to bind rhetoric more securely to the city while subtly loosening the bond between the audience and its beloved athletes.

It is clear, too, that Demosthenes' concern lies with the glory of the speech itself, for it is "what has been said (*rhēthē*)," that is rendered beautiful, *kalos,* by the kind listeners. Further, in the lines preceding this passage, Demosthenes specifies that this instructive call for goodwill is meant for those "outside the race," *exo tou genous,* implying that Athenians, by virtue of being Athenians, listen to *epitaphioi* with goodwill (*eunoia*).

Demosthenes' suggestion that the spectacle of the athletic contest is already imbued with the kind of honor that garners the viewers' approval is in line with Isocrates' treatment of the spectacle mentioned earlier in this chapter, when he observes that everyone present finds in the festival some aspect that produces a love of honor simply by virtue of the crowd's presence (*Panegyricus* 44). In other words, in the case of athletic performance, the honorable act requires only a gathering of witnesses in order to enter into the economy of glory (*kudos*)[11]—the honor is somehow internal to the competitive exhibition of speed and strength and is thus more passively accumulated through observation.

Demosthenes' move to link his rhetorical efforts to athletics therefore cuts at least two ways: first, it yokes the two endeavors together as means of producing honor, for he makes it clear that the athletic spectacle is the other accepted way to produce honor for the dead. Second, Demosthenes' account tacitly criticizes the spectacle of athletic performance, again along the lines of Isocrates' writing at the opening of *Panegyricus,* when he marvels at the disparity between the treatment of men with athletic prowess and those with the wisdom demanded by oratory (*Panegyricus* 1). Demosthenes' point diverges slightly, however. While Isocrates marvels that the spectacle of athletic display could be privileged over an art so deeply involved in the affairs of the city (i.e., rhetoric), Demosthenes more pointedly draws the audience into honor's fold, making listeners active participants in the circulation of honor, in that their very presence and their willingness to believe the orator's remarks on honor are necessary preconditions to the speech's success. In short, the crowd itself—its gathering—rather than the performing body of the athlete, becomes a rhetorical proof.

The work of honor-production is more dispersed in the case of rhetoric. Both orators therefore attempt to uplift their art in relation to athletics: Isocrates by extolling the virtues of orators in comparison to athletes, and Demosthenes by pointing out how much more rhetoric depends upon the spectators, and how much less on the ostentation "lavish" spending affords. The rhetoric of value for athletes depends on visible display, while the value for oratory depends on collective honor-seeking.

Yet another axis of relation between rhetoric and athletics emerges in Demosthenes' *Epitaphios:* the work of sight and sound in producing and circulating honor. Curiously, it is this very intimation that may just undermine Demosthenes' point. Toward the end of his speech, Demosthenes reflects that the war dead are no doubt "seated beside the gods" on the island of the blessed (*en makaron nēsois*) (34), and then goes on to clarify:

> For there is no sighting (*idōn*) or report (*apēggelken*) about them, yet the living we assume worthy of honors, and, basing our estimation on their fame, we believe them to succeed and lead the way to honor (*timōn*) there as well. (*Epitaphios* 34)

Here, then, besides rendering the honor of the dead a logical and temporal extension of the honor of the living, Demosthenes specifies the two registers on which the living are decided to be worthy of honor: through that which is seen and through that which is reported.

For the ancients, the visible tended to be the more reliable register, as Heraclitus writes, "the eyes are more exact witnesses than the ears" (DK 22 B101a). Further, as Vernant points out, *idein,* "to see," and *eidenai,* "to know," both derive from *eidos,* "appearance, visible aspect" (1995: 12). Thus, vision and knowledge were, in some ways, synonymous, and vision was considered somehow prior to knowledge. Still, though, sound and hearing mattered as well, for as Heraclitus also writes, "those things of which there is sight, hearing, knowledge (*opsis, akoē, mathēsis*): these are what I honor most (*protimeō*)" (DK 22 B55). Noteworthy here is the way in which *mathēsis* seems to build on sight and hearing, or at the very least, the grammatical parallel places them all on the same plane as Heraclitus' most privileged modalities of appearance.

There was, however, a profound distrust of these senses among poets and philosophers, for the eyes and ears as bodily instruments were thought to be inherently deceptive, never reaching the truth, *alētheia.* As Plato's Socrates quizzically puts it: "Have the sight and hearing of men any truth in them, or is it true, as the poets are always telling us, that we neither hear nor see anything accurately?" (*Phaedo* 65b). Socrates' question, significantly, appears in a lengthy discussion of the body as a hindrance (*empodion*) to pure knowledge or truth.

As Socrates puts it to his friend, "the corporeal is burdensome and heavy and earthly and visible (*baru, geōdes, horaton*)." It is the body, not the soul, that sees and is seen. When ethereal "pure" knowledge is the point of inquiry, when souls have to "contend" with the bodies by which they are "put in bondage (*katadeitai*)" (83d), the senses become difficult to bear. When, conversely, bodies contend with and observe other bodies, as in the case of funerals and festivals, the senses—especially, in this case, sight and the visible, hearing and sound—are the only available witnessing-tools.

It is noteworthy, too, that unlike Socrates, Heraclitus does not take recourse to a notion of "truth" per se but speaks instead of the equivalence among vision, hearing, and *mathēsis,* the production of knowledge.[12] Likewise, Demosthenes' imaginary extension of visible, reported, corporeal honor to the invisible world of the dead also calls upon Heraclitus' sight/sound/knowledge triad, thus helping to secure the logic of festive funerary practices: the "solemn honors owed the dead" are repaid to and by the *polis* through athletic and rhetorical performances, performances that reroute honor to what is seen, heard, and said.

Bodily Economies of Showing and Telling

Things get interesting when the seen, the heard, and the said enter into relation with each other. As modalities of appearance, seeing, hearing, and saying operate to produce honor much like fire and water work to produce flesh, as detailed via the Hippocratic texts and considered in chapter 4. That is, elements vary to produce particular qualities of differently valued honor. And it is Socrates, via passages in Plato and Xenophon, who helps illustrate this point.

The opening lines of Plato's *Republic* depict Socrates recounting firsthand the previous day's main activity: he went down to Athens' port, the Piraeus, to offer devotions to the goddess Bendis, for whom a new festival had just begun. Socrates' interest in the festival was straightforward: he "wanted to see" (*boulemenos theasasthai*) how it would turn out. He then reports that the Athenian procession was quite good, as was the show (*ephaineto*—literally "that which was brought to light") put on by the Thracians.

At first glance, Socrates' account depends entirely on the visual: he desired to see, and this is what he saw. The dialogue's frame thus demonstrates the way in which, as I have been suggesting, ancient festivals hinged on a logic of *epideixis*—a display, a demonstration, a showing forth, a making known. This list of lexical nuances for the word itself suggests the way in which a "showing" shades into "knowledge": just as in Heraclitus, "making visible" easily turns into "making known." Yet even in the passage from the *Republic,* the showing becomes immediately sutured to the telling, as Socrates narrates the festival's splendors: a telling reactualizes what Socrates saw.

The very term *epideixis* displays the necessary relation between showing and telling; for those who study rhetoric associate *epideixis* with a particular kind of speech, one of Aristotle's "big three"—epideictic, deliberative, forensic (*Rhetoric* 1.3.1–3). Still, *epideixis* primarily meant a material or bodily display, as when Thucydides employs the term to describe an Athenian naval expedition's "display of power" (*epideixis . . . tēs dunameōs;* 6.31.4), or when Xenophon uses the word to describe the beautiful Theodotē's display of her body (*Memorabilia* 3.11.2). But again, in these instances the display itself becomes manifest via discourse.

Xenophon's passage is worth considering in more detail, since Theodotē's posing prompts Socrates to interrogate the economy of *epideixis* at work, particularly with regard to two critical relationships under consideration here: seeing/hearing and performer/audience. Significantly, the section begins with a tale of her beauty, told to Socrates, who is found, as usual, in a thicket of friends. To the account he replies, "We must go and see (*theasomenous*) . . . for hearing a word is not as powerful as to examine closely (*katamathein*)." Here, Socrates seems to buttress Jay's point about the priority of vision over language.

Socrates' informant at once leads him to Theodotē's house, where, finding the woman posing for a painter, they looked on, *etheasanto.* This scene prompts the following exchange, with Socrates as the central speaker:

> "Ought we to have more gratitude to Theodotē for showing us her beauty (*to kallos heautēs epedeixen*), or she to us for looking (*etheasametha*)? Does the favor lie with her, if the display profits her more, or with us, if looking profits us more?"
>
> When someone answered that this was a fair way of putting it: "Therefore," he said, "she already benefits from our praise, and when we spread the news more, she will benefit even more; whereas we already desire to touch what we have seen, and we leave somewhat excited and will long for her when we depart. But out of this we become her attendants, and she the one we attend to (*therapeusthai*)."

Then Theodotē exclaimed, "By Zeus, if what you hold is so, of course I ought to be grateful to you for looking (*tēs theas*)." (3.11.2–3)

A subtle contradiction inheres between the lines in which Socrates feels impelled to see instead of hear and the logic of his economic assessment. Despite the fact that Socrates, like Heraclitus, gives priority to what is seen over what is heard, when he considers the benefits, the "telling" that follows the seeing becomes once again infused with value: "when we spread the news (*diangeilōmen*), she will profit yet more." Xenophon therefore presents a viewing sandwiched between two tellings, a chain of events, each enabling the next in turn: the telling ultimately infuses the seeing with a new value, since through words the moment of visibility can be reactualized to others not present. The passage suggests then that while vision may be more closely tied to knowledge, both vision and hearing/telling are, together, critical for the production of fame.[13]

Furthermore, viewers in this scenario are not passive recipients of the display and the knowledge it produces, but rather are credited with actualizing Theodotē's beauty, precisely by completing the reciprocal equation and making her display a display. As Demosthenes' treatment of the eulogy suggests, and as Simon Goldhill points out in his discussion of the term, quite simply, "*epideixis* requires an audience" (1999: 3). Both witnesses and the witnessed thus constitute the showing, and as evident both in Plato's *Republic* and in Xenophon's *Memorabilia,* the viewer and performer have a reciprocal, codependent relation. But it is the possibility of another, future audience that demarcates telling from seeing. Not only does discourse act to reactualize vision, but it disrupts vision's priority by bringing it forward both spatially (to other places) and temporally (into the future).

Further, the witness of a performance—be it artistic (as in the painting), dramatic, musical, athletic, poetic, or rhetorical—takes an active role in eliciting the display as well as in responding to it. Jeffrey Walker argues along these lines in his treatment of *epideixis* in rhetoric, invoking Aristotle's suggestion at *Rhetoric* 1.3.1358b that an epideictic audience member should be a *theōros,* "one who is to make observations (*theōriaia*) about what is praiseworthy, preferable, desirable or worthy of belief in the speaker's *logos*" (2000a: 9). That is, Walker goes on to argue, epideictic discourse demands an active evaluation and response. Evidence supporting this phenomenon may be found in the discussion of funeral orations above, in particular Menexenus' response to Aspasia's speech, as well as Lysias' contention that he is in contest with those who have gone before him.

Further, as Simon Goldhill puts it, *epideixis* is almost inevitably competitive, and as such "it necessarily triangulates competition through an audience" (1999: 3). In other words, the logic of display, enabled by the presence of a crowd of witnesses, works to provoke response but is also already structured as an agonistic response itself. To further delineate this epideictic agonism, however, it is necessary to examine more closely the dynamics of Greek vision and hearing in relation to spectacular display.

The Flames of Vision

As the Theodotē incident and the chapter's opening quote from Nietzsche both suggest, ancient epideictic logic is engendered by a model of vision radically different from the one that informs contemporary treatments of the spectacle.

In many contemporary accounts, the act of viewing becomes an almost violent/violating act of objectifying, insofar as it renders the bodies or things viewed as just that—things. But, as Goldhill points out in a rare and thorough discussion of the Xenophon passage, "the gaze, for Xenophon's Socrates, even—especially—when directed by a man at a beautiful woman, is not a unilinear process of objectification" (1998: 115). Contrary to the dominant contemporary notion of vision, that is, the Greek notion of sight, rather than demarcating subject and object, depends on a kind of exchange. As Socrates' economic question in the Xenophon passage above makes clear, the visible here relies on reciprocity, and both the spectators and Theodotē are active participants.

Such a perspective regarding vision is fueled by ancient theories of optics, which, as Froma I. Zeitlin points out, "hold that light emanates from the eyes as well as from the source of light" (1996: 189). Furthermore, this notion of vision requires a kind of reciprocity that also carries over into identity production. Zeitlin continues: "It is reciprocal too in social terms, in the relations between one self and another, because each party both sees and is seen by the other in the mutuality of vision" (189). Similarly, Ruth Padel discusses the eyes as a symbol for reciprocity, in the light of their "twin roles" as receptors and emitters (1992: 61–63).

Just as the ancient notion of vision clashes with our modern inter-pretation of it as simple objectification, it also disrupts more general as-sumptions contemporary Westerners hold about spectating. "To view" is not, in the Greek scheme, actively violent, nor is it conceived of as a passive, receptive act, a "taking in" of sorts. Greek eyes, rather, were thought to be connective organs, and in this regard, they were no dif-ferent from the hands in that they could reach out and grasp—and be grasped by—something or someone else. This connective function of vision is elucidated most saliently in Plato's *Timaeus*, where the title character, in his elaboration of the composition of human form, char-acterizes the organs of sight as "light-bearing eyes (*phōsphora ommata*)" (*Timaeus* 45b). According to Timaeus, the gods

> caused the pure fire within us . . . to issue forth through the eyes in a smooth dense stream . . . so whenever the light of day surrounds the stream, it flows from like to like, and joins together; one body of its own is constituted (*hen sōma oikeiōthen*) according to the direc-tion of the eyes it forms one kindred substance along the path of the eyes' vision, where the fire which streams from within collides with an obstructing object without. (*Timaeus* 45c)

In other words, the fiery eyes were thought to extend outward, to meet the flames issuing forth from things "outside," and in the min-gling of flames, in the joining of light, to comprise an altogether new body (*sōma*). As Vernant describes it, "there was, to explain vision, a sort of luminous arm-like tentacle, which through the eyes extended one's organism outside itself" (1995: 15). It is important to note, too, that within this theory of extramission (the notion that the eyes trans-mitted as well as received light rays), the meeting of flames—sight—happens between the seer and the seen; thus in *Timaeus*, attention is effectively shifted away from the seer and seen in order to emphasize the actualization of the new body that exists only on the line of vision, precisely through the encounter itself. It is this in-betweenness of vision that Zeitlin refers to as reciprocity and mutuality, and that prompts Jay to observe that the Greek notion of vision entailed "a certain participa-tory dimension in the visual process, a potential intertwining of viewer and viewed" (1993: 30).

As Vernant and Zeitlin intimate, it is precisely their intertwining that upends the very distinction between subject and object in theories of Greek optics. At times, too, the path of vision intermingles with other fluidlike substances such as that mediating, in-between force of *eros,* which, as Euripides writes in *Hippolytos,* "drips desire from the eyes" (525–26). It is no coincidence that *eros* is thought to draw substance from the eyes, as vision operates on a logic of seduction: Timaeus makes clear that the flames of vision are drawn together, like compelled toward like (*homoion pros homoion; Timaeus* 45c).

If, as Vernant contends, to see is to know, then the logic of vision — and by extension, knowledge — depends on a moment of seduction, on a movement outside the self, a mingling with the flames of the other. It could well be, then, that desirous honor, *timē,* like Euripides' notion of *erōs,* clung to the flames from the eyes, and was thereby transported from one to another, along the line composed by the fiery gaze/display construct. Such a view would account for the recursivity in Isocrates' account of the mutual distribution of the love of honor: "the spectators when they see the athlete exert themselves for their benefit, the athletes when they reflect that all the world is come to gaze upon them" (*Panegyricus* 44). The very structure of the spectacle stokes a love of honor between performers and spectators.

This self-overcoming mingling of appearances, further, is precisely why Nietzsche proclaims the Greeks profound in their very superficiality, for the seductive promise of mingling is what drew Greeks to festivals. An example of such seduction on the visual register can be found in Aristophanes' *Clouds,* when the nubial chorus proposes a visit to Athens:

Rainbearing maidens,
Let us visit the gleaming land of Pallas, to see the ravishing
   country
Of Cecrops with its fine men, gleaming . . .
Where ineffable rites are celebrated, where
The temple that receives initiates is thrown open during the pure
   mystic festival;
And where there are offerings to the heavenly host,
Temples with lofty roofs and statues,
Most holy processions for the Blessed Ones,
Well-garlanded victims for the gods, and feasts in all seasons;
And with spring comes the grace of Bromius,
The rivalry of melodious choruses
And the deep-toned music of pipes. (*Clouds* 299–314)

This passage emphasizes the seductive promise of the visual, and the way the visible makes known the ineffable. The first four lines present Athens, "ravishing" and distant, a glimmering location (*liparan pallados*) (a grammatical construction presented in parallel with "its fine men" [*euandron*]). The home of the Parthenon, the architectural *epideixis par excellence*,[14] is wholly other in its splendor, beckoning seductively: "Come. See." But, as this chapter has suggested, the beckoning does not stop at the level of the visual. In fact, vision is part of another kind of mingling: that with sounds and words. Festivals and funerals were far from mute, as evident in the *Clouds* passage, which ends with the sonorous quality of the City Dionysia festival, even invoking Dionysus' resounding epithet, Bromius, "The Noisy," and ending with reference to the competing sounds of singers and *aulos*-players. Certainly sights and sounds blend together in a festal context to flood the senses with overwhelming proof of the occasion's grandness.

Recall, too, that Nietzsche, in addition to "forms," which operate on the register of the visible, includes in the Greek "Olympus of appearance" tones and words. The sheer noise of celebration—the voices and pipes and applause reverberating through the city, and finally, the work of discourse—cannot be ignored in a diagram of the spectacle.

A Thunderous Crowd

In addition to the pipes and the mellifluous noises of choral efforts, onlookers themselves made a good deal of racket. Athenian audiences were a noisy, responsive lot, and evidence of their rowdiness abounds in ancient literature.

Pindar's *Olympian* 9 speaks of the victorious wrestler Epharmostos, who "passed through the ring of spectators to such great shouting / being young and fair and performing the fairest deeds" (*Ol.* 9.92–93). For Pindar, the sheer volume of noise—"such great shouting (*hossa bo*)"—stands as evidence of Epharmostos' beauty, *kalos*. Epharmostos, by virtue of his greatness, elicits the crowd's strong response, which in turn serves to support his performance and seal his honor.

The honor here—and this is a key point—is measured audibly, by the force and intensity of the noise: Pindar's poem serves as a sort of ancient applause-o-meter. Marked for its sheer volume, this spectator noise works affectively, penetrating Epharmostos' body far more than the regarding gaze of which it is a noisy reminder. The reverberating shouts, though, also work effectively, bespeaking honor, and propelling Epharmostos to his next honorable act, where he "made a marvelous appearance" at an Arkadian festival (line 96). The penetrative force of noise therefore operates in tandem with the visual, as a noisy reminder of the audience's thereness, the "live" in-person spectator, a necessary part of the structure of *theōrian,* the driving force of the festival.

Plato's Socrates, however, is compelled to dissect the joint affective/ effective quality of crowd response, this time in the context of rhetorical performance. After Socrates labels the populace the "chief kind of sophist," the interlocutor asks him when such a phenomenon occurs, and he replies:

> Whenever the multitude are seated together in assembly, in court-rooms, at the theater, in camp, or at any other public gathering of a crowd. With loud uproar they will make known their approval or censure, both in excess, producing constant uproar, calling aloud and clapping, the place together with the rocks themselves resounding and doubling the noise of censure and of praise. In the case of a young man speaking, how do you suppose the heart will hold back? What private teaching will enable him to withstand not being deluged by the current of praise and blame until he makes known whatever the crowd says is base or honorable, until he is ready to do as they do and be as they are? (*Republic* 492b–c)

Here, the affective quality of the noise, marked by the movement of the young performer's heart, *kardia,* becomes intensified by the very space of performance, as the surrounding topography effectively refracts and doubles the noise. The crowd, Socrates worries, has the capacity to drown out the speaker, to sweep him up in its frenzy, to ultimately take over. As with vision, then, noisemaking has its own kind of reciprocity: the tenor and volume produces a measurable feedback by which the performer might then become inspired (as with Pindar's Epharmostos) or drawn into another way of thinking (as with Socrates' rhetorical performer). Like music (as considered in the previous chapter), crowd noise marks a considerable affective/effective force within the performer/spectator relation.

It is important to note, too, that on the very basis of this affective feature of crowd noise, Pindar's noisy crowd signifies differently from the one Socrates' cites in the *Republic*. That is to say, while Pindar's crowd stands to mark Epharmostos' athletic honor and simultaneously reproduce it, the specto-auditors of rhetorical performance can serve to debase the speech (in the *Republic* description). This distinction between crowd effects in the two scenarios hinges on a body/*logos* divide: the athletic body may be productively subject to the crowd's din, but the rhetorical body (according to Socrates) must protect itself against a change of heart *via* the crowd's noisy invasion.

Feedback, though, already entails ongoing response, as both the athletic and rhetorical performer elicit responses while in the mode of responding; both inhabit a recursive *agōn*. Often, too, the noise of the audience works together with the words of the speaker to intensify the situation's agonistic dimension, as when Socrates, in a passage discussed in chapter 1, compares the effects of Protagoras' speech to the staggering strike of a "skillful boxer," as he was made "quite blind and dizzy with the effect of his words and their shouts of approval" (*Protagoras* 339e). The effect, then, of the listeners' spectacular din combined with Protagoras' discursive pummeling is almost entirely affective: the assault takes away Socrates' most rational of senses—his sight—leaving him groping for recovery, both of his rational bearings and his place in the exchange.

In this scenario, we can see the triangulation of competition through the audience at work in the logic of *epideixis*. Not only does the presence of the crowd enable the logic of agonistic display, the crowd constantly reminds performers of its active presence as it gathers and participates in the circulation of honor and shame through its pulsing, thunderous noise.

Protagoras is not the only place where Socrates aligns crowd with speaker and produces the economy of honor as an affective endeavor. In *Menexenus,* Socrates describes the affective response brought on by the performer(s), in this case, the commissioned funeral orators, who praise

> so well . . . with the beauty and variety of their diction, they bewitch our souls; and they praise the State at every turn, and commending those who died in the war and all our ancestors before and ourselves who are living still; so that I myself, Menexenus, when praised by them in this way I feel altogether ennobled, and every time I listen fascinated I regard myself to have become taller and nobler and more handsome on the spot. And I am generally accompanied by a number of strangers of the sort who listen along with me, to them I

become more majestic on the spot; for they also manifestly receive my impressions with regard both to me and to the rest of our City, believing it to be more marvelous than before, thanks to the persuasive eloquence of the speaker. (*Menexenus* 235a–b)

In this rather mocking account of the effects of public orations,[15] Socrates describes an appearance of honor through discourse. The "strangers" in the passage, those who have come along to listen, are not described as being persuaded as much as they simply *see* Socrates differently after the speech: Socrates has transformed, become taller, nobler, and better looking—in short, in the described scenario, he has become amplified.[16] Honor's circulation hinges on this discursive amplification, and in this passage, Socrates approximates the figural growth of Epharmostos in the Pindar passage described above, only here honor is put into circulation by the combination of the performer's persuasive eloquence and the listeners' response.

The stylistic effect Socrates seems to be describing here is what Aristotle calls *pro ommatōn poiein,* a phrase Kennedy translates literally as a "bringing before the eyes" (*Rhetoric* 3.10.4; 3.11.1).[17] When discussing this particular trope, Aristotle makes recourse to the language of vision, action, and time, arguing that "things should be seen as being done rather than as in the future" (3.10.6), or, most clearly, "I call those things 'before the eyes' that signify things engaged in an activity" (3.11.1).

As such, the phenomenon of "bringing before the eyes" is bound to *energeia,* a trope that suggests activity or, as Kennedy points out in a gloss of Aristotle's discussion of *the term,* also "actualization" or "vivification" (1991: 249 n. 133). Through *energeia,* then, "bringing before the eyes" animates the figure by infusing the person or thing under discussion with a kind of action and presentness; while Socrates' account to Menexenus above does not give a clear example, he is nonetheless describing the effects of this particular trope insofar as it "brought Socrates before the eyes" of the listener as "more majestic," the city "more marvelous."[18] Indeed, this trope, because it marks discursive visualization, the active force of language, stands as the trope of *epideixis,* the genre of display.

Perhaps the logic of the visible is epideictic's tightest enthymeme. Sutured both to the Presocratic logic of vision—seeing is knowing—and also to a bodily logic of motion (*energeia*) and emotion, the visual operates both through and in tandem with discourse as *logos* reproduces and circulates the visible. The circulation of the visual through discourse, though, happens quickly, at times stealthily, often unsettling its own economy.

Speech's Invisible Body

In his much-discussed encomium on Helen, the sophist Gorgias, in arguing that *logos* might be more culpable in Helen's actions than she herself, offers the following justification: "Speech is a powerful lord that with the smallest and most invisible body accomplished most godlike works. It can banish fear and remove grief and instill pleasure and enhance pity. I shall show how this is so" (*Helen* 8; trans. Kennedy [1980]).

This passage, often taken as a representative nugget of Gorgias' rhetorical theory, points to the *non*-visibility of discourse, speech's "smallest and most invisible body" (*smikrotatoiōi sōmati kai aphanestatoi*). Rhetorically, this passage refers back to the immediately preceding passage, in which Gorgias argues that Helen may have been seized by force: the body of Paris, it is implied, through brute strength may have overpowered the body of Helen. Similarly, speech has a body, albeit small and not immediately apparent. That is, it is endowed with its own brand of what Derrida, in a brief consideration of this passage, calls "furtive force" (1981: 116); *logos* has a peculiar capacity to produce material effects, as Derrida puts it, "to break in, to carry off, to seduce internally, to ravish invisibly" (116). Speech is a stealthy body, stalking visible bodies, becoming manifest through the motion it incites, through the bodies it affects or, to take recourse to Gorgias' language of speech as drug, through the bodies it inhabits.

Gorgias, the grand magician of words, is about to expose the wares of his stealthy art—to render visible his own invisible body. With the last line of the passage, "I shall show how this is so," Gorgias deploys the verb *deixō*, from *deiknumi*, which may be translated "bring to light, to render, to display," and which comes from the noun *deixis*, which has the force of both rhetorical proof in the Aristotelian sense and also anatomical demonstration. In other words, by anatomizing speech through his own oxymoronic "invisible body," Gorgias will render visible the way in which Helen might have been subject to the invisible body of speech.[19] Gorgias' proof is also his rebuttal.

In the realm of appearances, then, discourse unsettles the visible by inhabiting the paradoxical space between the invisible and the visible:

by producing visible effects through invisible, "furtive" force, and such force is enacted in discourse's ability to, quite simply, move.

A Rumor of *Kleos*

Following the widely considered opening scene of Plato's *Phaedrus*—the cloak scene made more famous by Derrida—the title character, when trying to coax Socrates into delivering a speech better than that of Lysias, issues a threat. If Socrates refuses to participate, Phaedrus swears by the plane tree beside them that he will never again deliver a speech for Socrates unless his request is heeded. In doing so, he deploys two separate verbs: *epideixein* and *exangelein*. That is, Phaedrus "will never display or report" to Socrates any other speeches.

The first verb he uses, from *epideixis,* we have encountered repeatedly. The second derives from the noun *exangelia,* "a making known," as in the case of a messenger (*angelos*) or an informant. Here *exangelia* indicates indirect discourse, a report of a speech—words about words. One might say that all of Plato's dialogues coalesce around such indirect reports, as characters move about and recount events just witnessed, whether a great speech or a spectacular festival. Such reports are predicated upon the movement of news, the spreading of words.

It is this capacity to spread through iteration,[20] a feature unique to discourse, that secures honor for spectacular performances. A passage from Pindar simultaneously invokes vision and movement to secure an important place for his songs. He sings:

> But as for me, while I illuminate that dear city
> With my fiery songs
> More swiftly than either a magnificent horse
> Or a winged ship
> I will send this announcement everywhere.
> (*Ol.* 9.21–25)

If considered alongside Greek theories of extramission—the emission of fire from objects that meets the flames issuing from the eyes—this passage merges poetic discourse itself into the light-giving aspects of the visible, as Pindar's songs "illuminate" the city. But these lines argue for discourse as "value-added," for he invokes the capacity of his songs to proliferate: faster than horses and ships carrying cargo, he sends his words everywhere, *panta.* So Pindar's hymns, through their combination of the visual and movement, are more effective than the visual alone—according, of course, to Pindar.

As Pindar's lines suggest, as has been demonstrated through Socrates' arguments about Theodotē, and as Demosthenes' diagram of the funeral oration points out, seeing is so inexorably bound with telling that together they constitute a double actualization—the witness, that is, actualizes the display and in momentary transformation becomes a bearer of news, a messenger newly endowed with discourse's capacity to relay, the second actualization. The witness/messenger thus makes a new display, effectively reintroducing the logic of *epideixis*. Speech's "invisible body," as Gorgias calls it, becomes manifest; the priority of the visible is disrupted.

And just as the gathering itself produces the display, so the capacity to hear most often entails the capacity to say or repeat—hence the etymological linkage between *kluō,* I hear, and its noun—*kleos*—"that which is heard, a report, a rumor." As Goldhill points out, the connotations of *kleos* inevitably gravitate toward glory, honor, and fame (1991: 69).

The same pattern of migration in meaning happens in regard to the other word for rumor, *phēmē,* the "common report, rumor, fame." As Sian Lewis demonstrates in her study of news in ancient Greece, rumors "were seen to spring up . . . and to travel unnaturally fast" (1996: 13). Again, the focus here is movement, but this movement of news, reputations, glory is detached from any source—in the case of *phēmē,* that is, the word travels so fast that it cannot keep track of its origins— the news exists, instead, as "common report"—"it is said."

Unhinged from its originary moment of visibility, news not only disrupts the priority of the visible, but it goes so far as to erase the moment of the visible, assuming an appearance all its own—this time in the guise of words. Rather than rendering *phēmē* dubious, though, its lack of origin exalted *phēmē* to the level of the divine. Thanks to the proliferative quality of speech, that is, the report takes on an *ēthos* and agency of its own, able to confer honor in a single iteration, over and over.

Aeschines' treatment of *phēmē* delineates its economy of rumorous honor: "a common report (*phēmē*) which is unerring does *of itself* spread abroad throughout the city" (*Against Timarchus* 1.127). Aeschines then goes on to note the fact that Athens and its forefathers "dedicated an altar to *phēmē* as one of the greatest gods" (1.128). In a reversal of the movement I have been tracing here, the discursive, *phēmē*, is thus translated into a spectacle, an altar marking the divine quality of rumor.

Unmoored from its origin, then, rumor takes on a divine quality through both its action and its style of movement. In the manner of Pindar's poems, more swiftly than horses or ships, rumor's invisible body thus confers honor untrackably, rendering visible through its invisible, furtive force. It is this dual capacity for rendering visible through iteration that places rhetoric so firmly in the structure of the ancient spectacle and allows it to mix in to different degrees with the visible.

At the heart of Isocrates' and Demosthenes' concern about athletics' priority over rhetoric, then, is the presumed priority of the visible over the articulable. While Isocrates overtly condemns the privileging of athletic displays over oratorical ones, he nonetheless upholds the collective, gathering force of the festival and the centrality of the athletes. Demosthenes differently worries the privilege of ostentation and the frenzied obsession with elaborate display of athletic contests and contrasts the active participation required of the audience by an orator with the sheer spectacle of athletic displays. Both nonetheless want to link their art to athletics by means of comparison, and both do so by describing an economy of honor circulation to which rhetoric is indispensable. Both, further, articulate such an economy by invoking the binding force of speech's invisible body.

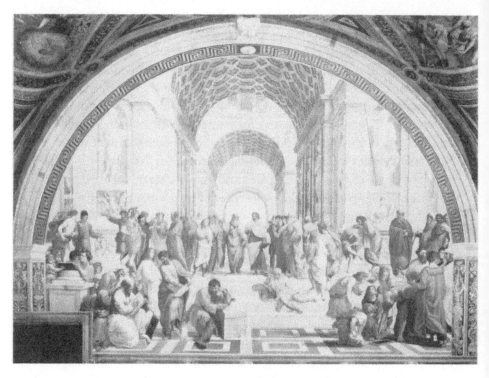

FIGURE C.1
"The School of Athens," Raphael, 1511. Vatican Museum.

Conclusion

Raphael's "School of Athens" (figure C.1) could stand on its own as this book's conclusion. Completed in 1511 and shown here in its restored form, the fresco presents an almost seamless blending of classical Greece with early modern Italy, as it simultaneously cites the flowering and the reflowering of the intellectual.

In the foreground, Heraclitus writes with his head perched on his hand and Euclid gives a geometry lesson; Raphael features himself in the painting as well as his contemporary, Michelangelo. And of course Plato and Aristotle, Greek philosophy's dynamic duo, enter at the painting's illuminated center, discoursing amidst a throng of followers.

The fresco further achieves its thematic blend by featuring architectural elements from both cultures: while the vaulted ceilings are reminiscent of the Roman basilica form revived during Raphael's era (Lieberman 1997: 71–76), the open-air quality of the background (note the visible sun and clouds) hearkens back to the quasi-outdoor space of the ancient Greek gymnasium. Art historians know that Raphael studied Vitruvius, the ancient scholar of architecture (Hall 1997: 5), and as Giovanni Bellori argues, an equally—if not more—suitable title for the painting would be "Gymnasium of Athens" (1997: 49).

Thus by simultaneously depicting the figures and contexts of both ancients and contemporaries, Raphael's "School of Athens" offers what art historian Ralph Lieberman calls "a glimpse into a world governed by reason, where civilized inquiry and enlightened discourse take place in a setting of appropriate grandeur and decorum" (1997: 64). In this way, the elaborate fresco renders what is probably the most widely held conception of classical Athens and its legacy: a high regard for cerebral activity and the development of the mind, an unabashed love of wisdom writ as ideas.

As such, the painting enthymematically tells the story of what began to happen as the fourth century came to a close. The painting tells, that is, how gymnasia became (and hence became remembered as) Athenian "schools" in the modern sense: how they sprouted tables and chairs, and how, moreover, when Aristotle died and passed on his school to his former student and assistant Theophrastus in 322, the Lyceum subsequently became home to an impressive library with holdings covering an array of subjects wider than that of any other philosophical school (Grayeff 1974: 78–81). Intellectual development thus took over as the gymnasium's foremost activity, and the gymnasium's legacy, like the legacy of the Greeks, became equated with Plato and Aristotle, with philosophy, with the development of the mind.[1]

Swathed in brightly colored garments, all the characters in the painting stand in sharp contrast to the naked unidentified statue with which this book began. The somato-centric culture of Greece remains submerged, unnamed, not unlike the shipwrecked bronze itself. Ancient *aretē,* that is, is remembered and reproduced not as Aristotle himself suggested, in the somatic form of *kalos kagathos,* but rather as the Great Mind, the possession of intellectual prowess. Forgotten is the early blending of bodily and intellectual training practices; gone are the considerations of rhythm, repetition, and response in education; and while the clusters of students around Socrates, Pythagoras, and Euclid suggest a gleaming hint of *sunousia* (a becoming by association) the figures and disciplines nonetheless receive more emphasis than do the dynamics and practices facilitated through teacher-student encounters.

In many ways, then, this book also stands as a response to the "Myth of the Mind" found in Raphael's painting, particularly the ways in which histories of rhetoric have been erected upon and hence have perpetuated that myth. This study instead has tried to historically produce the *agōn* of rhetoric as not just a "meeting of the minds," but rather as a full-on, whole body encounter between rhetor and rhetor or teacher and student, an art concerned with a deeply habituated, embodied, situated intelligence and sense of timing.

More specifically, this book begins to fill in Raphael's picture by considering ways athletics and rhetoric can be treated syncretically. The impulse to do so, I contend, comes from the ancient orators themselves —most notably Protagoras, Gorgias, Isocrates, Demosthenes, and even Plato. While rhetoric and athletics no doubt had their distinctive aims, they came together as arts of training and performance to help foster a generalized situational bodily knowledge mediated by *mētis* and *kairos*. Teachers of these twin arts, as Isocrates suggests, often drew on similar methods of what chapter 4 calls phusiopoietic production (friendship, erotics, and pain); shared the same architectural space; and fashioned their pedagogies around principles of movement (rhythm, repetition, and response).

But the convergence of these arts is not limited to training practices. As chapter 7 argues, the bodily knowledge yoking rhetoric and athletics functions on a macro-level as well—in terms of a widespread knowledge of bodies. Put differently, the kinds of productive, educative actions that occur on the level of the body—the mixing in of elements, the agonistic formation of flesh (as conceived by the Hippocratics)— are recapitulated on the level of culture, wherein bodies meet and mix in with bodies, be it in the context of the festival, the *agōn*, or the taking-in of a display, *epideixis*. Both bodily learning and bodily culture are shot through with desire and knowledge, often connectively transmitted through optical, aural, and tactile exchange.

Throughout this book, then, I have emphasized the sensual intensities of fifth- and fourth-century Athens: the reverberating *auloi*, the vibrant purple robes of orators and poets in competition, the deep thundering noise of a festival crowd, and oily, sandy skin rubbing on skin as wrestlers grappled in training or in competition. The depictions of bodies in the form of statues or on pottery help, too, to underscore a chiasmatic point more saliently than any amount of discursive repetition: ancient arts knew bodies, and their bodies knew art. The intermingling, mutually constitutive, agonistic practices of athletics and rhetoric, brought together at times by spectacular, uplifting festivals, at others by dark-toned, somber funerary rituals, were ultimately treated as bodily arts by the itinerant teachers of rhetoric who first approached these arts syncretically. Athletics and rhetoric thus came together as bodily arts that reinforced and perpetuated the lively culture of contact, movement, and sound so markedly Athenian.

Agonism These Days

As with many treatments of ancient history, especially those under-taken from the vantage point of contemporary rhetorical education, the question of "them" versus "us" permeates this study. While we would do well to bear in mind the productive styles of agonism developed by the ancients, such styles should be distinguished from today's "cross-fire" style of agonism, found most frequently in the pummeling style of cable television's debate shows, which would more aptly be described as instances of antagonism.[2]

This distinction between antagonism and agonism is one that has been consistently elided, as, for example, in Deborah Tannen's "Ago-nism in the Academy" (2000) When Tannen uses the term agonism to discuss the "ritual" of "scholarly attack" found everywhere in aca-demia—from reading groups to graduate student training to faculty meetings and printed scholarship—she seems to be complaining about what this study has termed *ant*agonism. While the ancient Greeks were no doubt practitioners of antagonism, or what Hesiod terms unpro-ductive strife—they went to war, they squashed each other publicly, rhetorically, and sometimes physically—ancient Athenians nonethe-less understood the distinction between spiteful, contentious battling and intense, productive exchange, and tended to prefer the latter to the former.

Agonism's potential for productive struggle is taken up by Susan Jar-ratt in an article on agonism and pedagogy (1991a). Here, Jarratt poses the question, "How might conflict be productive?" Her treatment of the *agōn,* by emphasizing the exchange that happens in classroom de-bates, moves toward the "gathering" notion of agonism put forth by the ancients and discussed at length in this book's first chapter. Consider-ing rhetoric as *agōn,* then—at least as it is formulated early on in this study—might help figure rhetorical education as itself a gathering—of issues, practices, bodies, values, differences—and a kairotic occasion for developing new and different but always careful responses.

If, as one of this study's main points contends, only the *agōn* can teach the *agōn,* it becomes even more necessary to distinguish what sorts of *agōnes* are able to operate productively. Antagonism, for instance—the attack-mode that Tannen finds distasteful and damaging—is rarely pro-ductive of anything but a puffed-up attacker and a squashed attackee. In contrast to this "whack-a-mole" style of interacting, the kind of agonism this study discusses and regards as productive would take the form of insistent questioning, intense engagement with the issue under consideration, and/or an exchange between colleagues. It might involve a protracted, variegated inhabiting, not unlike that exhibited by Demosthenes in his subterranean study (see chapter 6), a wrestler studying and imitating a *paidotribēs,* or the kind of engaged, sustained inquiry found in the best of academic monographs. Such prolonged engagement ensures that the resulting position (and disposition) is thorough, responsive, and—importantly—likely never finished. Instead, such engagement comes to be about the questing itself, questing for thinking, transforming, considering, and reconsidering: what many might consider learning.

Bodies and Teaching

How, then, might an analysis of sophistic rhetoric as bodily learning and practice hold relevance for contemporary rhetorical pedagogy? This question evokes another of this study's themes: that sophistic rhetoric is a bodily, habituated practice dependent upon rhythm, repetition, and response.

By considering bodies in the contexts of learning and performing, this study joins in with those who have become keen on the importance of the body, timing, and a flexible responsive intelligence. T. R. Johnson's *A Rhetoric of Pleasure* (2003), with its attention to desire, the visceral, and sound, does much to link teaching nowadays to theories of the body, both contemporary and ancient. Christine Pearson Casanave (2002), in her choice of the game metaphor for describing academic writing practices, implicitly acknowledges agonism's role in rhetorical education. Figuring writing as a game further enables Casanave to acknowledge the ways bodies think, as she discusses how "rules" become so deeply internalized as to become bodily (2002: 4).

The game analogy also allows a focus on situational learning, which connects back to this book's treatment of *mētis* and *kairos.* The importance of *mētis* and *kairos* in linking agonism, flexible intelligence, and bodily learning to contingencies of knowledge production can also be glimpsed in an ethnographic study of physicists by Elinor Ochs and Sally Jacoby (1997). The study, entitled "Down to the Wire," examines the changing modes of collaboration scientists employ as conference deadlines approach. Ochs and Jacoby demonstrate how changing time constraints as the conference draws near—what amounts to a question of *kairos*—bring to the fore questions about rhetoric, delivery, and expediency. Time as timing, or *kairos,* becomes a critical catalyst, eliciting different responses from the physicists to the situation, to each other, to the subject matter, to the field itself.

Ochs and Jacoby's rich data attend to bodily gestures alongside the question of timing and adaptability. While Ochs and Jacoby use a compendium of grammatical markers to indicate changes in volume, pitch, stress, and intonations of voice, they also use italics to indicate the physical gestures accompanying these vocal gestures. What results, effectively, is an account of bodily, scholarly engagement.

Consider, briefly, their rendering of a response from one of the physicists to a rehearsal of the upcoming conference paper:

> Ron: I have a problem. (*removes glasses*)
> *Miguel looks at Ron*
> *Ron lays glasses on table*
> With your talk,
> *Ron puts hand to forehead*
> *Miguel looks down.*
> Uh not with the physics in it, but with the lack of references to anybody else's work. (1997: 486)[3]

In tracking the physicists' kairotic shifts from discussing matters of physics to discussing matters of rhetoric, Ochs and Jacoby also document the agonistic struggle evident in their bodily demeanors and gestures. In short, evident in Ochs and Jacoby's transcripts is a cheironomic taxonomy. Further, as the physicists rehearse and discuss their performances, elements of training and performing converge to suggest that the physicists are keen on the *agōn*'s role in preparing for the *agōn* (the conference gathering, in this case). The shifting emphases, values, and guises are brought to the fore in Ochs and Jacoby's study as bodies are mixed in with physics and rhetoric—manner binds with matter as the physicists prepare for their performance.[4]

In many ways, these scholars are doing what anthropologist Paul Stoller argues is critical: "to incorporate into ethnographic works the sensuous body—its smells, tastes, textures, and sensations" (1997: xv). Stoller's more surprising goal, however, is to simultaneously "reawaken the scholar's body" (xvi), which he suggests has been slumbering away,

Rip Van Winkle–like, for centuries. Yet Ochs and Jacoby's account of the collaborating physicists would suggest otherwise.

At stake in all these studies is a point made variously by the likes of Judith Butler, Michel Foucault, N. Katherine Hayles, Elizabeth Grosz, and most notably, Pierre Bourdieu: knowledge-making habits and practices cannot be extricated from the body. Bodily knowledge is therefore a necessary and vital aspect of what scholars today are calling "intellectual work," a term used to indicate all the kinds of work we do as scholars and teachers.

Even as scholars begin to notice the body's role in learning and performing, the body nevertheless often seems far from the concerns of contemporary classrooms, as students squash their physical selves into sleek formica desk-chair combos, sitting upright for the duration of the class. Or worse, in the increasing move to large lecture classes, certain aspects of *sunousia* (the protracted associative pedagogy discussed in chapter 6) become a distant fantasy.

What's more, the arrival of distance education brings with it different physicalities of education. Such pedagogical conditions might risk producing a disconnectedness unfavorable for learning. Or perhaps large lectures and online courses enable different modes of pedagogy, those that emphasize modeling or impressing, for example. My concern here is not to diagnose these new phusiopoietic structures, but rather to bring the body to bear, so to speak, on these changes in the conditions of higher learning. If the ancient gymnasium, as suggested in chapter 5, provided a productive site for gathering, what styles of learning do classroom spaces and structures enable and foreclose? What sorts of sounds and sights infiltrate the areas devoted to learning? Such questions demand further study as phusiopoietic spaces continue to evolve and emerge. At stake in these particular questions, borne from this study, is a concern for the bodily learning that takes place regardless of the milieu in which training happens.

As this book argues, the body's centrality in learning and performing is something the ancients knew so well as to almost take for granted. Ancient rhetoricians and orators gleaned this lesson from athletic training and performance, after which they fashioned their art. This curious syncretism had important effects on rhetoric's development, as the nascent art came to share taxonomies, agonistic flair, conceptions of intelligence and time, pedagogical strategies, and cultural value with the already established and well-regarded athletic enterprise.

As I have been suggesting throughout this book, a return to the syncretic tradition of the Greeks refigures the long-accepted view depicted in Raphael's "School of Athens" by calling attention to rhetoric's status as a bodily art. Such attention to bodies as they learn, perform, and transform alters as well existing rhetorical practices, pedagogies, and histories.

Notes

INTRODUCTION

1. Perseus reading: Svoronos 1908: 26–27; Paris: Staïs 1910; Hermes: Gardner 1903.

2. Hermes Logios: Waldstein 1901; rhetor: von Mach 1903.

3. For a discussion of the translation of *aretē,* see chapter 1.

4. For a consideration of Isocrates' choice of term, see Poulakos 1997: 69–70; de Romilly 1992: 51–52.

5. See, e.g., Plato, *Republic* 402e.

CHAPTER 1

1. One might object to Vernant's observation that it was the gods that were anthropomorphic—i.e., that human form didn't imitate god-form, but vice versa. Vernant, however, is insistent:

> It is rather the reverse: in all its active aspects, in all the components of its physical and psychological dynamism, the human body reflects the divine model as the inexhaustible source of a vital energy when, for an instant, the brilliance of divinity happens to fall upon a mortal creature, illuminating him, as in a fleeting reflection, with a little of that splendor that always clothes the body of a god. (1989: 28)

2. Poetry, in fact, was the first art to call attention to language's visual capacity, as the old sophistic poet Simonides, according to Plutarch, placed poetry on the same plane as painting, calling "painting silent poetry and poetry painting that speaks" (*Glory of Athens* 3; see also Yates 1996: 28 and Lee 1967: 197; chapter 7 below).

3. Thanks to Jeffrey Walker for bringing this passage to my attention. Walker discusses the line in depth: 2000a: 205–6.

4. This line and the following lines from *Protagoras* represent my modifications of Lamb's translation.

5. Lamb translates *sunousia* and all its forms in this passage as "classes," thus marking the regular, somewhat formal structure of the interactions. But *sunousia* has a particular meaning suggesting a being together, a coming together, even a society (see chapter 6), and the emphasis is less on the formal structure suggested by "classes," and more on regular repeated association. By translating it "conversations," I have chosen to mark it as the latter.

6. Here Hippias engages in what might today be called a bit of "trash talking," the element of agonism *par excellence,* wherein competitors goad each other by proclaiming their own superiority. While Hippias may come across as a pompous man who wants merely to call attention to himself, I would suggest that the goading, like that of Gorgias, functions to provoke others to enter into the struggle by issuing a challenge, hence falling under Hesiod's category of productive strife, or true agonism.

7. Among others, Aristotle cites Gorgias's *Olympic Discourse,* a speech given at the Olympic Games (*Rhetoric* 1414b). Whether this was an official contest is hard to know; note, however, the use of *agōnizesthai* in the Hippias passage, along with the two instances (discussed below) of the *agōn* root used in relation to Gorgias.

8. At the time of Ctesiphon's motion, Aeschines protested its illegality on two counts: one, that the constitution forbade the crowning of a public official until after his term was over, and two, that it also restricted the location of said crowning to the Pnyx (Ctesiphon proposed to issue the crown in the Theater of Dionysius). Demosthenes was still in office as superintendent of the Festival Fund.

9. Also at stake, of course, were the political alliances that lay at the very heart of the rivalry between Demosthenes and Aeschines; whereas Aeschines was known to collude with Philip of Macedon, Demosthenes vigorously promoted an anti-Macedonian policy (Vince and Vince 1953: 12–13; for more on Athens' volatile politics in the late fourth century BCE, see Sealey 1993; Harris 1995).

10. The reason for the delay is unknown; see Vince and Vince 1953: 3; Sealey 1993: 201; Adams 1948: 306.

11. As in his speech *Against Timarchus* 176.

12. Many scholars place the *logoi* part of the title as implied (c.f. Mirhady and Too 2000: 240 n. 64); Hermann (1995: 104) offers the participle form, *kataballontōn,* "throwing down," as an alternative title. This suggestion is supported by fragments from Sextus (DK B1).

13. See Diogenes Laertius, *Lives* 3.4.

14. See chapter 5.

15. C.f. Hermann's extensive treatment (1995) of wrestling metaphors in *Theatetus.*

16. Here I follow Dover (1968: lvii–lix), Kastely (1997a), and O'Regan (1992) in employing the *kreitton–hetton* distinction, as opposed to the *dikaios–adikaios* (just and unjust) distinction.

17. For more in-depth discussions of the *kreitton–hetton* contrast, see O'Regan 1992: 89–105, Nussbaum 1980, and Kastely 1997a.

18. For a thorough and useful examination of the *agōn* in Aristophanic comedy, see Timothy Long, who suggests that "the paradox in the use of the *agōn* in Aristophanes is not that he goes out of his way to introduce the *agōn* . . . but that, having introduced a form eminently adapted to persuasion, he never allows the outcome of the *agōn* to dictate the course of the action in the rest of the play" (Long 1972: 286). O'Regan (1992) also offers a close analysis of the *agōn* in the *Clouds.*

CHAPTER 2

1. For an in-depth consideration of *thumos,* especially as related to *psychē* and *nous,* see Padel 1992: 28–30.

2. *Iliad:* 1.311, 1.440, 3.200, 3.216, 3.268, 4.329, 4.349, 10.148, 10.382, 10.400, 10.423, 10.488, 10.554, 14.82, 19.154, 19.215, 23.709, 23.755; *Odyssey:* 2.173, 4.763, 5.214, 7.207, 7.240, 7.302, 8.152, 8.165, 8.412, 8.463, 8.474, 8.486, 9.1, 11.354, 11.377, 13.311, 13.382, 13.416, 14.191, 14.390, 14.439, 15.380, 16.201, 17.16, 17.192, 17.353, 17.453, 18.14, 18.51, 18.124, 18.312, 18.337, 18.365, 19.41, 19.70, 19.106, 19.220, 19.261, 19.335, 19.382, 19.499, 19.554, 19.582, 19.585, 20.36, 20.168, 20.183, 20.220, 21.404, 22.1, 22.34, 22.60, 22.150, 22.170, 22.320, 22.371, 22.390, 22.430, 22.490, 23.129, 23.247, 23.263, 24.302, 24.330, 24.356, 24.406.

3. For a reading of the entire *Odyssey* as an *agōn* between Athena and Odysseus, see Clay 1983.

4. See chapter 1's discussion of the particular connection between wrestling and sophistic rhetoric as arts where the weaker can hold forth.

5. Pierre Bourdieu makes much of the idea of *hexis* as it connects to thought as an embodied practice. As Bourdieu describes it, "bodily *hexis* is political mythology realized, *em-bodied,* turned into a permanent disposition, a durable way of standing, speaking, walking, and thereby of feeling and thinking" (1990: 70). Here Bourdieu makes an important connection between movement and thought by way of *hexis,* which articulates thought *as* movement.

6. For more on rumor in relation to rhetoric and the circulation of honor, see chapter 7.

7. Chapters 4 and 6 will discuss this productive force of "practice" as central to sophistic training.

CHAPTER 3

1. For the usefulness of *kairos* in contemporary rhetoric, see Kinneavy 1991 and 2002 and Carter 1988. James S. Baumlin offers an in-depth discussion (1984) of the concept's relationship to *prepon,* or decorum. More recently, Colin Gifford Brooke (2000) articulates *kairos* as a key concept for the posthuman. More philological treatments of *kairos* include those of William H. Race (1982), Richard Broxton Onians (1951: 343–48), and J. R. Wilson (1980 and 1981). For important and rarely cited (at least in rhetorical scholarship) philosophical work on *kai-*

ros's relationship to *chronos*, see John E. Smith (1969). Also, Carolyn Miller (1992) has made good use of the concept in relation to technology and the rhetoric of science.

2. Richard Leo Enos has recently documented the way *chronos* and *kairos* came together in his fascinating study of the ancient *klepsydra* or water clock—the device often used to measure (and limit) the duration of speeches (2002: 77–78). Such clocks, as Enos puts it, provided "some degree of temporal reckoning" (80) and functioned as a constraining force on speakers. Enos's article might be said to recall an ancient genealogy, for while *kairos* is usually distinguished from *chronos*, as it is here and in Quintilian's *Institutio Oratoria* (2.6.26), Kairos's status as the youngest son of Zeus makes him the grandson of Chronos.

3. The difference is accentual: a circumflex over the iota (*kaîros*) versus an accent grave on the last syllable (*kairós*). Onians' connection between the "aperture" reading of *kairós* and the weaving term is as follows: "*kaîros* was evidently in some sense the warp or something in the warp, something to do with the 'parting' of its threads. It is generally taken to mean the row of thrums which draw the odd warp-threads away from the even, making in the warp a triangular opening, a series of triangles, together forming a passage for the woof" (1951: 346).

4. Onians (1951: 340) argues convincingly for taking *peirata* as weaving and following the metaphor through; hence, his translation: "If you speak to the point and pithily—with much matter in a little space, with the texture of your speech close, well knit—less cavil follows."

5. This line of inquiry inspired a spate of articles on the rhetorical situation, most notably by Lloyd Bitzer (1968), Richard Vatz (1974), and Kathleen Hall Jamieson (1974).

6. See Atwill's compelling comparison between Pierre Bourdieu's notion of an embodied art and ancient notions of habituation (1998: 58–59). An examination of athletic *kairos* extends Atwill's point beyond embodied learning to bodily performance, and the sophistic approach to rhetoric through a kairotic body.

7. For a fascinating comparative account of the body in Greek medicine, see Kuriyama (1999), whose treatment of the body's pulsations and Chinese and Greek approaches to learning through different models of touch and expression, together with her mention of the *iatrosophistos* (doctor-sophist), during the Second sophistic, "when ties between medicine, philosophy, and rhetoric became tighter than ever" (1999: 68), holds fascinating implications for thinking of medicine and rhetoric as bodily arts.

8. Two key early works provide important background for this argument: Jacqueline de Romilly's work (1975) on rhetoric and magic, and E. R. Dodds's *The Greeks and the Irrational* (1951: 179–206).

9. I have no reason to believe that this version of *kairos* counters Consigny's per se; rather, it teases out what he takes as implicit in the *agōn*.

10. Elsewhere, I term this version of *kairos* "invention in the middle," detailing a kairotic model of rhetorical invention that troubles any clear-cut subject/object distinction (Hawhee 2002).

11. Hyde (1921: 177ff.) discusses the use of wings to indicate motion in ancient reliefs and sculptures, a now well-established observation.

12. The epigram's word is *didaskaliēn*—the accusative, objectival form of *didaskalia*.

13. In addition to those scholars mentioned previously, on this general point, see Jarratt 1991b: xv, 11; Guthrie 1971: 272; Untersteiner 1954: 110; Enos 1993: 83; Schiappa 1999: 73–74.

14. See, in particular, Stanford's chapter "Speech and Music" (1967: 27–48). Many thanks to Richard Enos for bringing this study to my attention.

15. For an important early work delineating the Gorgianic figures and examining their invention, see Robertson 1893.

16. This contagion model of language is elaborated usefully by Richard Doyle in the context of discourse in the biological sciences: "the transmission, passage, and communicability of language, therefore, become something other than an affair of meaning or information; they become something more like ballistics or contagion, the transmission and repetition of an effect across bodies of discourse and across bodies" (1997: 5). T. R. Johnson, too, usefully considers Gorgias in terms of "the contagion of pleasure" (2003: 3).

CHAPTER 4

1. So-called by Jacqueline de Romilly (1992: 15). For a detailed treatment of rhetoric as *technē*, see Janet Atwill's *Rhetoric Reclaimed: Aristotle and the Liberal Arts Tradition* (1998).

2. Precisely what the ancient elements were and how they fit into humoral doctrine varies among ancient authors. For more on ancient elements, see G. E. R. Lloyd's "Hot and Cold, the Wet and Dry in Early Greek Thought" (1964) and his *Early Greek Science* (1970: 57–61).

3. The Hippocratic author takes care to include the soul as, like the body, comprising these two elements (1.6.1).

4. For an excellent discussion of nature's relationship to culture in Presocratic thought, see John J. Winkler's *Constraints of Desire* (1990: 22). William Arthur Heidel offers an exhaustive early treatment (1910) of the various dimensions of *phusis*, also with special attention to Presocratic thought.

5. For a discussion of Archaic lyric as a culturally significant practice, especially in terms of rhetorical sensibilities, see Jeffrey Walker 2000a: 139–53.

6. For a more thorough consideration of how music relates to the rhythm of training, see chapter 6.

7. For more on *kairos* as bridging active and passive and thus disrupting agency, see my "Kairotic Encounters" (2002).

8. In *Chaosmosis,* Felix Guattari discusses Francisco Varela's distinction between "'allopoietic' machines which produce something other than themselves, and 'autopoietic' machines which engender and specify their own organisation and limits" (1995: 39) in the context of subject production and the machinic assemblages constituted between institutional and technical machines and humans.

9. This view of friendship approximates that of Derrida, wherein friendship involves entrusting oneself to the other ("I entrust myself, without measure, to the other. I entrust myself to him more than to myself, he is in me before me and more than me" [1997: 195]).

10. For friendship as contract, see Konstan 1997: 14, 29; see also Too 2000.

11. For an extensive treatment of flogging as punishment in the context of athletics and athletic training, see Crowther 1988.

12. For a general discussion of pain and asceticism in Antiquity, see Malina 1995.

13. It is the educative context on which I will focus; for a broader cultural study of ancient erotics, see Foucault's *Use of Pleasure* (1990) and *Care of the Self* (1988), as well as K. J. Dover's *Greek Homosexuality* (1978) and David Halperin's *One Hundred Years of Homosexuality* (1990).

14. Several Platonic dialogues suggest seduction goes on in the gymnasium, as does Aristophanes' *Clouds*. Calame offers a thorough discussion of erotics in the gymnasium (1999: 101–9). See also Dover 1978: 54–55.

15. *Erastēs* is used to denote the privileged position in both man-woman and man-boy relations. See Calame 1999: 19–23, 98–109, 186–91 and Dover 1978: 16–17 for a discussion of these terms. In *Use of Pleasure*, Michel Foucault also offers a useful elaboration of the *erastēs* and the *eromenos* and their respective roles in the erotic economy (1990: 196–97).

16. It is important to bear in mind, however, that the dialogue narrates only an ideal; it should not necessarily be taken to describe normative practices. David Halperin, arguing this point rather convincingly (and humorously), writes "it is wrong . . . to imply that Greek men made love to their boys with a copy of Plato's *Phaedrus* firmly tucked under one arm for easy consultation" (1990: 59).

CHAPTER 5

1. The third was the Cynosarges, originally designated for the training of young boys with only one parent from Athens and one from elsewhere (Gardiner 1910: 468). The facility later became the school of the Cynics.

2. Anon., *Life of Isocrates* (in Westermann 1845).

3. Much has been written on the difference between the palaestra and the gymnasium. "Palaestra" usually refers to an enclosed architectural space and is often part of a larger complex called the "gymnasium," a term which actually refers to the grounds—outdoor courts (Kyle 1987; Gardiner 1910; Beck 1964; Marrou 1956).

4. "Stones of Athens" is a term used by R. A. Wycherley (1978) to refer to the anthropological data offered up by archaeological remains.

5. For a useful discussion of the *peripatos* and the philosophical school named after it, see Lynch 1972: 74–77, and Wycherley 1961. For a thorough treatment of the evolution of the architectural structure of the Greek gymnasium and its connection to Roman baths, see Delormé 1960. For a more recent consideration of ancient baths, see Fagan 1999.

6. Donald Kyle's discussion of the *nothoi*'s association with the Cynosarges works through the contested evidence thoroughly and convincingly (1987: 88–92).

7. The logic behind the law, which is dubiously attributed to Solon, is supposedly a concern about teachers being alone with boys and in the dark.

8. These features of the Academy and the Lyceum were regarded as exceptional in antiquity (Glass 1967: 81).

9. See chapter 1 for a discussion of Socrates' description of the brothers as pankratiasts.

CHAPTER 6

1. The *aulos*, often translated "flute," is in fact more of an oboelike instrument, or a clarinet. Many scholars find the translation as "flute" objectionable (see Schlesinger 1939: xvii; Anderson 1966: 8), so I will leave it untranslated. For a stunning history of the instrument's material production and contribution to ancient musical theory, see Kathleen Schlesinger, *The Greek Aulos* (1939).

2. While I certainly do not want to conflate Archaic and Classical practices, I follow recent scholars such as Mark Griffith, who counters Marrou (1956) and Jaeger (1967) by arguing for more continuity in educational practices from the Archaic to the Hellenistic period (see Griffith 2001: 23 n. 2).

3. Because of my focus on athletic and rhetorical training, I will restrict my consideration of music to music in education—as provider of rhythm and mode—rather than on education in music, about which Aristotle and Plato both have a good deal to say (e.g., *Republic* 376d–403; *Politics,* Book 8).

4. For more on Damon's influence on Aristotle and Plato's theories of music, see Barker 1989: 316–17. For a discussion of the connections among *katharsis, pathos,* and musical modes, see Jeffrey Walker's "*Pathos* and *Katharsis* in 'Aristotelian' Rhetoric" (2000b).

5. For an extended meditation on music and the production of difference, see Gilles Deleuze and Felix Guattari's chapter, "1837: Of the Refrain" in *A Thousand Plateaus* (1987).

6. The source text here is Jüthner's rendering of the fragmented Greek manuscript (1969).

7. For a useful consideration of Theognis's relation to young Kyrnos, see Walker 2000a: 145–46.

8. See also Aristophanes' *Clouds,* where *Kreitton* gives a detailed account of the "old" style of education, elaborating principles of deportment, and the ways boys were instructed to sit and stand in the gymnasium.

9. Both Aristotle's and Aeschines' observations about bodily reading bring to mind Judith Butler's widely invoked notion of performativity, where gender becomes a "stylized repetition of acts" (1990: 140): as pointed out earlier, the bodies of Greek athletes—and rhetors, for that matter—were stylized as masculine; hence Aristotle and Aeschines offer a window onto the ancient production of masculinity as a bodily practice.

10. For a striking case of how in the early nineteenth century the concept of *cheironomia* became an art in and of itself, complete with its own compendium of bodily gestures, see Gilbert Austin's *Chironomia* (1966).

11. This passage and subsequent excerpts from Plutarch are translations adapted from Perrin.

CHAPTER 7

1. For a consideration of the intersections between drama and athletics, see Larmour 1999.

2. According to Neils (1992b), festival activities occupied a total of 120 days.

3. See Burkert 1985: 225–27. The Attic calendar begins with the *Hekatombaion,* a month named after the festival in Apollo's honor; this is followed by *Metageitnion* and *Boedromion,* which mark, respectively, a neighborhood festival and a festival of Apollo the Helper, respectively; then *Pyanopsion,* the boiling of beans, etc. For a thorough treatment of the relation between the festival year and the political (conciliar or prytany) year in Athens, see Meritt 1961.

4. According to the *Athenian Constitution,* the Nine Archons "also elect by lot ten men as Stewards of the Games, one from each tribe, who when passed as qualified hold office for four years, and administer the procession of the Pana-thenaic Festival, and the contest in music, the gymnastic contests and the horse-race, and have the Robe made, and in conjunction with the Council have the vases made, and assign the olive-oil to the competitors" (*Athenian Constitution* 60.1; trans. Rackham).

5. Credit for a version of this phrasing must go to Simon Goldhill ("democracy repeatedly made a spectacle of itself" [1999: 9]).

6. For a case for there being two *peploi* instead of one, see Barber 1992: 114 and Mansfield 1995, from which Barber cites evidence to make this point.

7. According to Kyle, the tenuous but conventional date for the reorganization of the Panathenaia is 566. It is also at this point that athletic contests were intro-duced (1992: 80), though the Panathenaic festival was by no means the first fes-tival to incorporate athletic games; rather, most festivals sprung from the games themselves.

8. Another crossover might be the poetic lamentation, *threnos.* Kennedy (1980) claims that the funeral oration derives from the *threnos,* but Loraux argues vigor-ously against such a claim, asserting rather that the funeral oration depended on Athens' *rejection* of the *threnos* (1986: 44). For an account of the funeral oration's communicative rhetorical functions, see Ochs 1993.

9. Willis's claim is quite straightforward: "Homer's games for Patroclus in *Iliad* 23, then, are by no means the prototype of the funeral games described in the other epics of the Cycle, but rather the culmination of a long tradition of the treat-ment of *athla* in epic or rhapsodic literature" (1941: 394).

10. Aristotle writes that it was the duty of the *polemarchos,* who presided over war, to organize these *epitaphios agones* (*Ath. Con.* 58.1).

11. Credit for the phrase "economy of *kudos*" goes to Leslie Kurke, whose

work provides an in-depth elaboration of such an economy. See her *Traffic of Praise* (1991) and the more recent *Coins, Bodies, Games, and Gold* (1999).

12. Of course, this marks out an important distinction between the concerns of the Presocratic and the Socratic philosophers regarding truth and knowledge.

13. It bears mentioning, too, that Socrates does not consider the painter in this economy of exchange. Wouldn't the resulting painting of Theodotē, like the news of her beauty, also serve as a tribute?

14. Richard Sennett (1994) offers a compelling description of Athenian architecture, with particular focus on the Parthenon, in his treatment of nakedness in Greek society.

15. For a thorough consideration of Plato's critique of funeral orations in *Menexenus,* see Loraux 1986: 267–70.

16. For a description of the rhetorical topic of amplification (*auxēsis*), see Aristotle, *Rhetoric* 1.9.39.

17. For an account of "bringing-before-the-eyes" see Newman 2002. While Newman's work bristles at the association of the concept with *energeia,* her conclusion that "bringing before the eyes" is about perceptive capacity nonetheless buttresses the discussion here (2002: 3, 5, 12).

18. George Kennedy, in the headnote to his chapter 11, discusses the characteristic Aristotelian emphasis on the visual, noting how, through this stylistic device, "the hearer sees something in a different way" (1980: 248).

19. See chapter 3 for a more in-depth consideration of Gorgias's encomium.

20. Of course the point about iteration is a long-standing one made by Plato in *Phaedrus* and elaborated by Derrida (1981; 1988). Still, both emphasize writing's ability to iterate in the absence of the speaker; neither emphasizes the speed of movement rumor suggests.

CONCLUSION

1. For an account of rhetorical education in this later period, one that, like my study, resists the Great Mind narrative, see Gleason 1995. And for the influence of Greece and Rome on Egyptian education, see Cribiore 2001.

2. Sharon Crowley and I try to make this distinction between contemporary and ancient rhetoric when we suggest that calling these shouting matches or instances of bullying "rhetoric" would be an unfortunate misnomer (2004: 1–5).

3. For the purposes of clarity I have removed the grammatical documentation accompanying this transcript. To view it, along with the key, see the original article.

4. As mentioned in the introduction, the body is explicitly foregrounded as well by Paul Prior and Jodie Shipka (2003), who trace out the complex and multilayered processes and spaces of literate activity by attending to questions of bodily movement as a necessary component to rhetorical invention. Questions of technology often lead researchers back to the body as well. Other ethnographers focusing on the body, Cynthia Selfe and Gail Hawisher (forthcoming), in their longitudinal study of literacy and technology, raise critical questions about the

body's role in learning and relating to technology. Christina Haas, too, focuses on issues of materiality and the body in her study of the use of technology (1996). Both these projects are in line with N. Katherine Hayles' insistence on keeping questions of the body and materiality at the fore of work on technology (1999). For two more noteworthy and compelling treatments of technology, materiality, and bodies, see Richard Doyle's new *Wetwares* (2003) and David Gunkel's "What's the Matter with Books?" (forthcoming).

Works Cited

Adams, Charles Darwin. 1948 (1919). "Introduction." In *The Speeches of Aeschines*. Greek text ed. and trans. Charles Darwin Adams. Cambridge, MA: Harvard University Press: 305–7.

Anderson, Warren D. 1966. *Ethos and Education in Greek Music*. Cambridge, MA: Harvard University Press.

Atwill, Janet M. 1998. *Rhetoric Reclaimed: Aristotle and the Liberal Arts Tradition*. Ithaca: Cornell University Press.

Austin, Gilbert. 1966. *Chironomia; or, a Treatise on Rhetorical Delivery*, ed. Mary Margaret Robb and Lester Thonssen. Carbondale: Southern Illinois University Press.

Barber, E. J. W. 1992. "The Peplos of Athena." In Neils 1992a: 103–17.

Barker, Andrew. 1984, 1989. *Greek Musical Writings*. 2 vols. New York: Cambridge University Press.

Baumlin, James S. 1984. "Decorum, *Kairos*, and the 'New' Rhetoric," *Pre/Text* 5.3–4: 171–83.

Beck, A. G. 1964. *Greek Education, 450–350 B.C.* London: Methuen.

Bellori, Giovanni Pietro. 1997. "The Image of the Ancient *Gymnasium of Athens*, or *Philosophy*." In *Raphael's School of Athens*, ed. Marcia Hall. Cambridge: Cambridge University Press: 48–56.

Bethe, E. 1907. "De dorische Knabenliebe: Ihre Ethic und Ihre Idee." *Rheinisches Museum für Philologie* 62: 438–75.

Bitzer, Lloyd F. 1968. "The Rhetorical Situation." *Philosophy and Rhetoric* 1.1: 1–14.

Bourdieu, Pierre. 1977. *Outline of a Theory for Practice*. Trans. Richard Nice. New York: Cambridge University Press.

———. 1990. *The Logic of Practice*. Trans. Richard Nice. Stanford: Stanford University Press.

Bremmer, J. M. 1990. "Adolescents, *Symposion*, and Pederasty." In *Sympotica. A Symposium on the* Symposion, ed. Oswyn Murray. Oxford: Oxford University Press: 135–48.

Brooke, Collin Gifford. 2000. "Forgetting to Be (Post)Human: Media and Memory in a Kairotic Age." *jac* 20.4 (fall): 775–95.

Bryant, Joseph M. 1996. *Moral Codes and Social Structure in Ancient Greece: A Sociology of Greek Ethics from Homer to the Epicureans and Stoics*. Albany: State University of New York Press.

Burkert, Walter. 1985. *Greek Religion*. Trans. John Raffan. Cambridge, MA: Harvard University Press.

Butler, Judith. 1990. *Gender Trouble: Feminism and the Subversion of Identity*. New York: Routledge.

Calame, Claude. 1999. *The Poetics of Eros in Ancient Greece*. Trans. Janet Lloyd. Princeton: Princeton University Press.

Carter, Michael. 1988. "*Stasis* and *Kairos:* Principles of Social Construction in Classical Rhetoric." *Rhetoric Review* 7.1: 97–111.

Casanave, Christine Pearson. 2002. *Writing Games: Multicultural Case Studies of Academic Literacy Practices in Higher Education*. Mahwah, NJ: Lawrence Erlbaum Associates.

Cheville, Julia. 2001. *Minding the Body: What Student Athletes Know about Learning*. Portsmouth, NH: Heinemann.

Clay, Jenny. 1983. *The Wrath of Athena: Gods and Men in the* Odyssey. Princeton: Princeton University Press.

Cohen, David. 1991. *Law, Sexuality, and Society: The Enforcement of Morals in Classical Athens*. Cambridge: Cambridge University Press.

Consigny, Scott. 2001. *Gorgias: Sophist and Artist*. Columbia: University of South Carolina Press.

Cook, A. B. 1965. *Zeus: A Study in Ancient Religion*, vol. 2. New York: Biblo and Tannen.

Cribiore, Raffaella. 2001. *Gymnastics of the Mind: Greek Education in Hellenistic and Roman Egypt*. Princeton: Princeton University Press.

Crowley, Sharon, and Debra Hawhee. 2004. *Ancient Rhetorics for Contemporary Students*. New York: Pearson Education.

Crowley, Sharon, and Jack Selzer, eds. 1999. *Rhetorical Bodies*. Madison: University of Wisconsin Press.

Crowther, Nigel B. 1985. "Male Beauty Contests in Greece: The *Euandria* and *Euexia*." *L'Antiquité classique* 54: 285–91.

———. 1988. "Flogging as Punishment in the Ancient Games." *Nikephoros* 11: 51–82.

———. 1990. *Logic of Sense*. Trans. Mark Lester with Charles Stivale. New York: Columbia University Press.

Deleuze, Gilles, and Felix Guattari. 1987. *A Thousand Plateaus: Capitalism and Schizophrenia*. Minneapolis: University of Minnesota Press.

Delormé, Jean. 1960. *Gymnasion: Étude sur les monuments consacrés a l'éducation en Grèce*. Paris: Bibliotèque des Écoles françaises d'Athènes et de Rome.

Derrida, Jacques. 1981. "Plato's Pharmacy." In *Dissemination*. Trans. Barbara Johnson. Chicago: University of Chicago Press: 63–171.

———. 1988. "Signature, Event, Context." In *Limited, Inc.* Evanston, IL: North-western University Press: 1–23.

———. 1997. *Politics of Friendship.* Trans. George Collins. London: Verso.

Detienne, Marcel, and Jean-Pierre Vernant. 1978. *Cunning Intelligence in Greek Culture and Society.* Trans. Janet Lloyd. Atlantic Highlands: Humanities Press, Inc.

Devereaux, George. 1967. "Greek Pseudo-Homosexuality and the 'Greek Miracle.'" *Symbolae Osloenses* 42: 69–92.

DK = Hermann Diels and Walther Kranz, *Die Fragmente der Vorsokratiker: Griechisch und Deutsch.* 3 vols. Berlin: Weidman, 1906–1910.

Dodds, E. R. 1951. *The Greeks and the Irrational.* Berkeley: University of California Press.

Dover, K. J. 1968. *Aristophanes' Clouds.* Oxford: Clarendon Press.

———. *Greek Homosexuality.* 1978. Cambridge, MA: Harvard University Press.

Doyle, Richard. 1997. *On beyond Living: The Rhetorical Transformations of the Life Sciences.* Stanford: Stanford University Press.

———. 2003. *Wetwares: Experiments in Postvital Living.* Minneapolis: University of Minnesota Press.

Enos, Richard Leo. 1993. *Greek Rhetoric before Aristotle.* Prospect Heights: Waveland Press.

———. 2002. "Inventional Constraints on the Technographers of Ancient Athens: A Study of *Kairos.*" In Sipiora and Baumlin 2002: 77–88.

Fagan, Garrett G. 1999. *Bathing in Public in the Roman World.* Ann Arbor: University of Michigan Press.

Forbes, Clarence. 1945. "Expanded Uses of the Greek Gymnasium." *Classical Philology* 40: 32–42.

Foucault, Michel. 1979. *Discipline and Punish: The Birth of the Prison.* Trans. Alan Sheridan. New York: Vintage.

———. 1988. *The Care of the Self: The History of Sexuality,* vol. 3. Trans. Robert Hurley. 3 vols. New York: Vintage.

———. 1990. *The Use of Pleasure: The History of Sexuality,* vol. 2. Trans. Robert Hurley. 3 vols. New York: Vintage.

Freeman, Kenneth J. 1969. *Schools of Hellas.* New York: Teachers College Press.

Gardiner, Edward Norman. 1905. "Wrestling." *Journal of Hellenic Studies* 25: 14–31.

———. 1910. *Greek Athletic Sports and Festivals.* London: Macmillan.

———. 1967. *Athletics of the Ancient World.* Oxford: Clarendon Press.

Gardner, Ernest. 1903. "The Bronze Statue from Cerigotto." *Journal of Hellenic Studies* 23: 152–56.

Gentili, Bruno. 1988. *Poetry and Its Public in Ancient Greece: From Homer to the Fifth Century.* Baltimore: Johns Hopkins University Press.

Glass, Stephen. 1967. "Palaistra and Gymnasium in Greek Architecture" (Ph.D. dissertation, University of Pennsylvania).

Gleason, Maud W. 1995. *Making Men: Sophists and Self-Presentation in Ancient Rome.* Princeton: Princeton University Press.

Goettling, C. W., ed. and comment. 1828. *Hesiodi Carmini.* Leipzig: Teubner.

Goldhill, Simon. 1991. *The Poet's Voice: Essays on Poetics and Greek Literature.* Cambridge: Cambridge University Press.

———. 1998. "The Seductions of the Gaze: Socrates and His Girlfriends." In *Kosmos: Essays in Order, Conflict, and Community in Classical Athens,* ed. Paul Cartledge, Paul Millett, and Sitta von Reden. New York: Cambridge University Press: 105–24.

———. 1999. "Programme Notes." In *Performance Culture and Athenian Democracy,* ed. Simon Goldhill and Robin Osborne. New York: Cambridge University Press: 1–29.

Graham, J. D. P. 1979. *An Introduction to Human Pharmacology.* Oxford: Oxford University Press.

Grayeff, Felix. 1974. *Aristotle and His School: An Inquiry into the History of the Peripatos with a Commentary on* Metaphysics *Zeta, Eta, Lambda, and Theta.* New York: Barnes and Noble.

Griffith, Mark. 2001. "Public and Private in Early Greek Institutions of Education." In *Education in Greek and Roman Antiquity,* ed. Yun Lee Too. Boston: Brill Press: 23–84.

Guarducci, M. 1966. "Divinità fauste nell'antica Veliea." *La Parola del Passato: Rivista di Studi Antichi* 108: 279–94.

Guattari, Felix. 1995. *Chaosmosis: An Ethico-Aesthetic Paradigm.* Trans. Paul Bains and Julian Pefanis. Bloomington: Indiana University Press.

Gunkel, David. Forthcoming. "What's the Matter with Books?" *Configurations* 10 (winter).

Guthrie, W. K. C. 1971. *The Sophists.* Cambridge: Cambridge University Press.

Haas, Christina. 1996. *Writing Technology: Studies on the Materiality of Literature.* Mahwah, NJ: Lawrence Erlbaum Associates.

Hall, Marcia. 1997. "Introduction." In *Raphael's School of Athens,* ed. Marcia Hall. Cambridge: Cambridge University Press: 1–47.

Halperin, David. 1990. *One Hundred Years of Homosexuality: And Other Essays on Greek Love.* New York: Routledge.

Halperin, David, John J. Winkler, and Froma I. Zeitlin. 1990. "Preface." In *Before Sexuality: The Construction of Erotic Experience in the Ancient Greek World,* ed. John J. Winkler, David Halperin, and Froma I. Zeitlin. Princeton: Princeton University Press: xv–xvi.

Harris, Edward M. 1995. *Aeschines and Athenian Politics.* New York: Oxford University Press.

Harris, Harold Arthur. 1966. *Greek Athletes and Athletics.* Bloomington: Indiana University Press.

Havelock, Eric. 1986. *The Muse Learns to Write: Reflections on Orality and Literacy from Antiquity to the Present.* New Haven: Yale University Press.

Hawhee, Debra. 2002. "Kairotic Encounters." In *Perspectives on Rhetorical Invention,* ed. Janet M. Atwill and Janice M. Lauer. Knoxville: University of Tennessee Press: 16–35.

Hayles, N. Katherine. 1999. *How We Became Posthuman: Virtual Bodies in Cybernetics, Literature, and Informatics.* Chicago: University of Chicago Press.

Heidel, W. A. 1910. *"Peri Phuseos:* A Study of the Conception of Nature among the pre-Socratics." *Proceedings of the American Academy of Arts and Sciences* 45: 77–133.

Hermann, Fritz Gregor. 1995. "Wrestling Metaphors in Plato's *Theatetus." Nikephoros* 8: 77–109.

Hyde, Walter Woodburn. 1921. *Olympic Victor Monuments and Greek Athletic Art.* Washington: Carnegie Institute of Washington.

Jaeger, Werner. 1967. *Paideia,* vol. 1. Trans. Gilbert Highet. 2nd ed. 3 vols. Oxford: Oxford University Press.

Jamieson, Kathleen Hall. 1974. "Generic Constraints and the Rhetorical Situation." *Philosophy and Rhetoric* 6.3: 162–70.

Jarratt, Susan. 1991a. "Feminism and Composition: The Case for Conflict." In *Contending with Words,* ed. Patricia Harkin and John Schilb. New York: Modern Language Association: 105–23.

———. 1991b. *Re-Reading the Sophists: Classical Rhetoric Refigured.* Carbondale: Southern Illinois University Press.

Jay, Martin. 1993. *Downcast Eyes: The Denigration of Vision in Twentieth-Century French Thought.* Berkeley: University of California Press.

Johnson, T. R. 2003. *A Rhetoric of Pleasure: Prose Style and Today's Composition Classroom.* Portsmouth, NH: Heinemann.

Johnstone, Christopher Lyle. 2001. "Communicating in Classical Contexts: The Centrality of Delivery." *Quarterly Journal of Speech* 87.2: 121–43.

Jones, W. H. S. 1953 (1931). *Hippocrates.* Cambridge, MA: Harvard University Press.

Jüthner, Julius. 1969. "Die Schriften der Paidotriben." In *Philostratos über Gymnastik.* Amsterdam: Grüner: 26–30.

Kastely, James L. 1997a. *"The Clouds:* Aristophanic Comedy and Democratic Education." *Rhetoric Society Quarterly* 27.4: 25–46.

———. 1997b. *Rethinking the Rhetorical Tradition: From Plato to Postmodernism.* New Haven: Yale University Press.

Kenakin, Terry. 1993. *Pharmacologic Analysis of Drug-Receptor Interaction.* New York: Raven.

Kennedy, George A. 1980. *Classical Rhetoric and Its Christian and Secular Tradition from Ancient to Modern Times.* 2nd ed. Chapel Hill: University of North Carolina Press.

———, trans. 1991. *Aristotle on Rhetoric: A Theory of Civic Discourse.* New York: Oxford University Press.

Kinneavy, James. 1991. *"Kairos:* A Neglected Concept in Classical Rhetoric." In *Landmark Essays on Rhetorical Invention in Writing,* ed. Richard E. Young and Yameng Liu. Davis: Hermagoras Press.

———. 2002. *"Kairos* in Classical and Modern Rhetorical Theory." In Sipiora and Baumlin 2002: 58–76.

Konstan, David. 1997. *Friendship in the Classical World.* New York: Cambridge University Press.

Kuriyama, Shigehisa. 1999. *The Expressiveness of the Body and the Divergence of Greek and Chinese Medicine.* New York: Zone.

Kurke, Leslie. 1991. *The Traffic in Praise: Pindar and the Poetics of Social Economy.* Ithaca: Cornell University Press.

———. 1999. *Coins, Bodies, Games, and Gold: The Politics of Meaning in Archaic Greece.* Princeton: Princeton University Press.

Kyle, Donald G. 1987. *Athletics in Ancient Athens.* Leiden: Brill.

———. 1992. "The Panathenaic Games: Sacred and Civic Athletics." In Neils 1992a: 77–102.

Lamb, W. R. M., trans. 1932. "Lysis." In *Plato,* Lysis, Symposium, Gorgias. Cambridge, MA: Harvard University Press.

———, trans. 1937. "Euthydemus." In *Plato,* Protagoras, Meno, Euthydemus. Cambridge, MA: Harvard University Press.

Landels, John. 1998. *Music in Ancient Greece and Rome.* New York: Routledge.

Larmour, David H. J. 1999. *Stage and Stadium: Drama and Athletics in Ancient Greece.* Hildesheim: Weidmann.

Lee, Rensselaer W. 1967. Ut Pictura Poesis *: The Humanistic Theory of Painting.* New York: Norton.

Lewis, Sian. 1996. *News and Society in Ancient Greece.* Chapel Hill: University of North Carolina Press.

Lieberman, Ralph E. 1997. "The Architectural Background." In *Raphael's School of Athens,* ed. Marcia Hall. Cambridge: Cambridge University Press: 64–84.

Lloyd, G. E. R. 1964. "Hot and Cold, Wet and Dry in Early Greek Thought." *Journal of Hellenic Studies* 84: 92–106.

———. 1970. *Early Greek Science: Thales to Aristotle.* New York: Norton.

Long, Timothy. 1972. "Persuasion and the Aristophanic Agon." *Transactions and Proceedings of the American Philological Association* 103: 285–99.

Loraux, Nicole. 1986. *The Invention of Athens: The Funeral Oration in the Classical City.* Trans. Alan Sheridan. Cambridge, MA: Harvard University Press.

Lynch, John Patrick. 1972. *Aristotle's School: A Study of a Greek Educational Institution.* Berkeley: University of California Press.

Mach, Edmund von. 1903. *Greek Sculpture: Its Spirit and Principles.* Boston: Ginn and Company.

Malina, Bruce J. 1995. "Pain, Power, and Personhood: Ascetic Behavior in the Ancient Mediterranean." In *Asceticism,* ed. Vincent L. Wimbush and Richard Valantasis. New York: Oxford University Press: 162–77.

Mansfield, John M. 1985. "The Robe of Athena and the Panathenaic Peplos" (Ph.D. dissertation, University of California at Berkeley).

Marrou, H. I. 1956. *History of Education in Antiquity.* Trans. George Lamb. New York: Sheed and Ward.

Meritt, Benjamin D. 1961. *The Athenian Year.* Berkeley: University of California Press.

Miller, Carolyn. 1992. "Kairos in the Rhetoric of Science." In *A Rhetoric of Doing: Essays on Written Discourse in Honor of James L. Kinneavy,* ed. Roger Cherry et al. Carbondale: Southern Illinois University Press: 310–37.

Mirhady, David C., and Yun Lee Too, eds. and trans. 2000. *Isocrates* I. Austin: University of Texas Press.

Mirhady, David C., Terry Papillon, and Yun Lee Too. 2000. "Introduction." In *Isocrates* I, ed. David C. Mirhady and Yun Lee Too. Austin: University of Texas Press: 1–11.

Muckelbauer, John. 2001. "Sophistic Travel: Inheriting the Simulacrum through Plato's 'The Sophist.'" *Philosophy and Rhetoric* 34: 225–44.

Murnaghan, Sheila. 1987. *Disguise and Recognition in the* Odyssey. Princeton: Princeton University Press.

Neils, Jenifer, ed. 1992a. *Goddess and* Polis: *The Panathenaic Festival in Ancient Athens*. Princeton: Princeton University Press.

———. 1992b. "The Panathenaia: An Introduction." In Neils 1992a: 13–27.

Newman, Sara. 2002. "Aristotle's Notion of 'Bringing-before-the-Eyes': Its Contribution to Aristotelian and Contemporary Conceptualizations of Metaphor, Style, and Audience." *Rhetorica* 20 (winter): 1–23.

Nietzsche, Friedrich. 1974a. *The Gay Science*. Trans. Walter Kaufmann. New York: Random House.

———. 1974b. "Homer's Contest." In *Early Greek Philosophy and Other Essays*. Trans. Maximillian A. Mugge. New York: Gordon Press.

Norlin, George, ed. and trans. 1982. *Isocrates* II. Cambridge: Cambridge University Press.

North, Helen. 1966. *Sophrosyne: Self-Knowledge and Self-Restraint in Greek Literature*. Ithaca: Cornell University Press.

Nussbaum, Martha. 1980. "Aristophanes and Socrates on Learning Practical Wisdom." *Yale Classical Studies* 26: 43–97.

Ochs, Donovan J. 1993. *Consolatory Rhetoric: Grief, Symbol, and Ritual in the Greco-Roman Era*. Columbia: University of South Carolina Press.

Ochs, Elinor, and Sally Jacoby. 1997. "Down to the Wire: The Cultural Clock of Physicists and the Discourse of Consensus." *Language and Society* 26.4: 479–506.

Onians, Richard Broxton. 1951. *The Origins of European Thought about the Body, the Mind, the Soul, the World, Time, and Fate*. Cambridge: Cambridge University Press.

O'Regan, Daphne. *Rhetoric, Comedy, and the Violence of Language in Aristophanes' Clouds*. New York: Oxford University Press, 1992.

Padel, Ruth. 1992. *In and Out of the Mind: Greek Images of the Tragic Self*. Princeton: Princeton University Press.

Paley, F. A. 1883. *The Epics of Hesiod*. London: Whittaker and Company.

Parke, H. W. 1977. *Festivals of the Athenians*. Ithaca: Cornell University Press.

Poliakoff, Michael. 1987. *Combat Sports in the Ancient World: Competition, Violence, and Culture*. New Haven: Yale University Press.

Porter, James I. 1999. "Introduction." In *Constructions of the Classical Body,* ed. James I. Porter. Ann Arbor: University of Michigan Press: 1–18.

Poulakos, John. 1995. *Sophistical Rhetoric in Classical Greece,* ed. Thomas W. Benson. Columbia: University of South Carolina Press.

Poulakos, Takis. 1997. *Speaking for the Polis: Isocrates' Rhetorical Education.* Columbia: University of South Carolina Press.

Prior, Paul, and Jodie Shipka. 2003. "Chronotopic Lamination: Tracing the Contours of Literate Activity." In *Writing Selves/Writing Society: Research from an Activity Perspective,* ed. Charles Bazerman and David R. Russell. Fort Collins, CO: WAC Clearinghouse Books, e-books: 180–238. (Available at *http://wac .colostate.edu/books/selves_societies/*)

Pucci, Pietro. 1987. *Odysseus Polutropos: Intertextual Readings in the* Odyssey *and the* Iliad. Ithaca: Cornell University Press.

Race, William H. 1981. "*Kairos* in Greek Drama." *Transactions and Proceedings of the American Philological Association* 111: 197–213.

Rackham, H., trans. 1935. *Aristotle,* Athenian Constitution. Cambridge, MA: Harvard University Press.

Redfield, James. 1994. *Nature and Culture in the* Iliad: *The Tragedy of Hector.* Durham: Duke University Press.

Robertson, John C. 1893. *The Gorgianic Figures in Early Greek Prose.* Baltimore: Friedenwald Company.

Roller, Lynn. 1981. "Funeral Games in Greek Art." *American Journal of Archaeology* 85: 107–9.

Romilly, Jacqueline de. 1975. *Magic and Rhetoric in Ancient Greece.* Cambridge, MA: Harvard University Press.

———. 1992. *The Great Sophists in Periclean Athens.* Oxford: Clarendon Press.

Russell, Donald, trans. 2001. *Quintilian,* The Orator's Education. Cambridge, MA: Harvard University Press.

Schein, Seth L. 1984. *The Mortal Hero: An Introduction to Homer's* Iliad. Berkeley: University of California Press.

Schiappa, Edward. 1991. "An Examination and Exculpation of the Composition Style of Gorgias of Leontini." *Pre/Text* 12.3–4: 237–57.

———. 1999. *The Beginnings of Rhetorical Theory in Classical Greece.* New Haven: Yale University Press.

Schlesinger, Kathleen. 1939. *The Greek Aulos: A Study of Its Mechanism and of Its Relation to the Modal System of Ancient Greek Music.* London: Methuen.

Sealey, Raphael. 1993. *Demosthenes and His Time: A Study in Defeat.* New York: Oxford University Press.

Segal, Charles P. 1972. "Gorgias and the Psychology of the Logos." *Harvard Studies in Classical Philology* 66: 99–155.

Selfe, Cynthia L., and Gail E. Hawisher. Forthcoming. *Literate Lives in the Information Age: Stories from the United States.* Mahwah, NJ: Erlbaum.

Sennett, Richard. 1994. *Flesh and Stone: The Body and the City in Western Civilization.* New York: Norton.

Shorey, P. 1909. "Physis, Melete, Epistem." *Transactions and Proceedings of the American Philological Association* 40: 185–201.

Sipiora, Phillip, and James S. Baumlin, eds. 2002. *Rhetoric and* Kairos: *Essays in History, Theory, and Praxis.* Albany: State University of New York Press.

Sirc, Geoffrey. 2002. *English Composition as a Happening.* Logan: Utah State University Press.

Smith, Bromley. 1921. "Gorgias: A Study of Oratorical Style." *Quarterly Journal of Speech Education* 7: 335–39.

Smith, John E. 1969. "Time, Times, and the 'Right Time': *Chronos* and *Kairos.*" *The Nionist* 53: 1–13.

Staïs, V. 1910. *Marbres et bronzes du Musé National d'Athènes.* Athens: Sakellarios.

Stanford, W. B. 1967. *The Sound of Greek: Studies in Greek Theory and Practice of Euphony.* Berkeley: University of California Press.

Stewart, A. F. 1978. "Lysippan Studies, 1: The Only Creator of Beauty." *American Journal of Archaeology* 82: 163–71.

Stewart, Douglas J. 1976. *The Disguised Guest: Rank, Role, and Identity in the* Odyssey. Lewisburg: Bucknell University Press.

Stoller, Paul. 1997. *Sensuous Scholarship.* Philadelphia: University of Pennsylvania Press.

Sullivan, Dale. 1992. "Kairos and the Rhetoric of Belief." *Quarterly Journal of Speech* 78: 317–32.

Sutton, E. W., and H. Rackham, trans. 1942. *Cicero,* de Oratore. Cambridge, MA: Harvard University Press.

Svoronos, J. N. 1908–1937. *Das Athener National Museum.* 6 vols. Athens: W. Barth.

Tannen, Deborah. 2000. "Agonism in the Academy: Surviving Higher Learning's Argument Culture." *Chronicle of Higher Education* 31 (March): B7–B8.

Thompson, James G. 1994. "The Agora: An Ancient Greek Sports Center." *Canadian Journal of History of Sport* 25.2 (December): 21–30.

Too, Yun Lee. 2001. "Introduction: Writing the History of Ancient Education." In *Education in Greek and Roman Antiquity,* ed. Yun Lee Too. Boston: Brill Press: 1–21.

———. 2000. *The Pedagogical Contract: The Economies of Teaching and Learning in the Ancient World.* Ann Arbor: University of Michigan Press.

Travlos, John. 1980. *Pictorial Dictionary of Ancient Athens.* New York: Hacker.

Untersteiner, Mario. 1954. *The Sophists.* Trans. Kathleen Freeman. Oxford: Blackwell.

Vatz, Richard E. 1974. "The Myth of the Rhetorical Situation." *Philosophy and Rhetoric* 6.3: 154–61.

Vernant, Jean Pierre. 1989. "Dim Body, Dazzling Body." In *Fragments for a History of the Human Body,* vol. 1, ed. Michel Feher. New York: Urzone: 18–47.

———. 1995. "Introduction." *The Greeks,* ed. Jean-Pierre Vernant; trans. Charles Lambert and Teresa Lavender Fagan. Chicago: University of Chicago Press: 1–22.

———. "One . . . Two . . . Three: *Eros.*" 1990. In *Before Sexuality: The Construction of Erotic Experience in the Ancient Greek World,* ed. John J. Winkler, David M. Halperin, and Froma I. Zeitlin. Princeton: Princeton University Press: 465–78.

———. 1983. *Myth and Thought among the Greeks.* Trans. Paul Kegan. London: Routledge.

Vince, C. A., and J. A. Vince. 1952 (1926). "Introduction to the *De Corona.*" In *Demosthenes* II, ed. and trans. C. A. Vince and J. A. Vince. Cambridge, MA: Harvard University Press.

Vitruvius. 1960. *The Ten Books on Architecture.* Trans. Morris Hicky Morgan. New York: Dover.

Waldstein, Charles. 1901. "Recently Discovered Greek Masterpieces." *Monthly Review* 3 (June): 110–27.

Walker, Jeffrey. 2000a. *Rhetorics and Poetry in Antiquity.* New York: Oxford University Press.

———. 2000b. "*Pathos* and *Katharsis* in 'Aristotelian' Rhetoric: Some Implications." In *Rereading Aristotle's Rhetoric,* ed. Alan Gros and Arthur Walzer. Carbondale: Southern Illinois University Press: 74–92.

Warry, J. G. 1962. *Greek Aesthetic Theory.* New York: Barnes and Noble.

Welch, Kathleen E. 1999. *Electric Rhetoric: Classical Rhetoric, Oralism, and a New Literacy.* Cambridge, MA: MIT Press.

West, M. L., ed. 1966. *Theogony.* Oxford: Clarendon Press.

Westermann, Anton, ed. 1845. *Biographoi vitarum scriptores graeci minores.* Brunsvigae: G. Westermann Publishers.

White, Eric Charles. 1987. *Kaironomia: On the Will-to-Invent.* Ithaca: Cornell University Press.

Willis, William Hailey. 1941. "Athletic Contests in the Epic." *Transactions and Proceedings of the American Philological Association* 72: 392–417.

Wilson, John R. 1980. "KAIROS as 'Due Measure'." *Glotta* 58: 177–204.

———. 1981. "KAIROS as 'Profit'." *Classical Quarterly* 31: 418–20.

Winkler, John J. 1990. *The Constraints of Desire.* New York: Routledge.

Wright, M. A. 1981. *Empedocles: The Extant Fragments.* New Haven: Yale University Press.

Wycherley, R. E. 1961. "Peripatos: The Athenian Philosophical Scene, I." *Greece and Rome* 8: 152–63.

———. 1978. *The Stones of Athens.* Princeton: Princeton University Press.

Yates, Francis A. 1966. *The Art of Memory.* Chicago: University of Chicago Press.

Zeitlin, Froma I. 1996. *Playing the Other: Gender and Society in Classical Greek Literature.* Chicago: University of Chicago Press.

Index

Academy. *See* gymnasium, Academy
actualization, 183
Aeschines
    Against Ctesiphon, 31–33, 198n9
    Against Timarchus, 4, 186, 198n11
    use of athletics, 30–36
    versus Demosthenes, 198n8
Aesop, 55
affect, music and, 140
agathos (goodness), 17, 19–20
agōn, 11, 13, 155, 182
    aretē and, 17–19, 24
    in Aristophanes' *Clouds,* 39–42,
        199n18
    bodies and, 15
    eristics and, 25
    flesh and, 90–91
    as gathering, 15–16, 28
    in Greek culture, 15
    kairos and, 12, 69–70, 73, 76, 200n9
    Odyssey and, 199n3
    performance and, 28
    response and, 19
    versus *athlios,* 15
agōnes, logon, 27–30
agonism, 192–193
    as bodily concept, 31
    cultural value of, 6
    Gorgias and, 29, 198n7
    learning and, 8, 156

Nietzsche on, 16
    pharmacology and, 26–27
    "questing" and, 28
    response and, 26
    rhetoric and, 16–17
    sophists and, 28–30, 37–39
    training and, 13, 154–155
    trash-talking and, 198n6
agora, 15, 111, 113–114
allopoiesis, 100
antagonism, 27, 192
Antikythera, Youth of, 2–3
apodyterion (undressing room), 117–118,
    123–124, 127–128, 131
    scenes from, 125–126 figs. 5.6–5.9
Apollo, 21
Archaic education, 4, 39–43, 96–98, 151,
    203n2
    depictions of, 133, 134 figs. 6.1, 6.2
archery, 67
architecture, of gymnasia, 112, 114, 116–
    118, 119–121 figs. 5.1–5.5, 128–129
aretē, 4, 6, 11, 165
    action and, 17
    agōn and, 17–19
    athletics and, 13, 30
    as bodily phenomenon, 17–18,
        21–22
    characteristics of, 21
    the gods and, 20–21

Walker, Jeffrey, 82, 197n3, 201n5,
203nn4,7
on *epideixis*, 176
on *meletē*, 146
on the octopus, 56
Rhetoric and Poetics in Antiquity, 8
Warry, J. G., 139–141
water, as bodily element, 90, 93
weaving, 67
Welch, Kathleen, 7
West, M. L., 49
White, Eric, 77
Willis, William Haley, 168, 204n9
Wilson, J. R., 199n1
Winkler, John J., 8, 105–107, 201n4

wrestlers
depicted, 143 fig. 6.6
as figures of *mētis*, 46, 55
wrestling
and body type, 20
kairos and, 84
rhetoric and, 34–39
treatise, 142
Wright, M. A., 58

Xenophon
Memorabilia, 167, 175
Symposium, 106

Zeitlin, Froma I., 177